Jenna Barbosa does just a phenomenal job of making grace feel attainable and life change possible. She uses her counseling background to make each chapter relatable and "chewable." *Tenacious Grace* is a great and easy read.

> —**Matt Bartig,** Lead Pastor at NorthRoad Church

Tenacious Grace is for every person who has ever suffered through both the struggle and shame of compulsive emotional eating. Jenna's authentic storytelling reveals the victory we can all experience in all the areas that seek to hold us captive. In fact, her broader focus on setting the reader free from all forms of idolatry makes this a must read. I can't get this book and its additional resources into the hands of my loved ones fast enough!

> —**Jayne Patton,** Founder of Altered Ministries

Don't think for a second that this book is only about food and therefore pass on reading it. That would be a huge mistake! Sure, now I'm going to look at why I run to Velveeta Shells & Cheese instead of a grilled chicken salad after a stressful day—and I should. But my biggest takeaways throughout the book were the powerful practical and spiritual wisdom I am now armed with.

Jenna has a beautiful way of captivating you throughout the entire book with her humility and personal testimonies with food. Take the Tenacious Grace journey with her! You'll be glad you did.

> —**Christy Boulware,** Founder and President of Fearless Women

Jenna Barbosa has written a gem with *Tenacious Grace*. Unlike other books that address eating disorders or weight loss, Jenna helps readers dig deep into the "why" of unhealthy eating. This is a must-read for anyone who has ever struggled with their relationship with food and wants to be set free from the grip of food addiction.

> —**Angie Allen,** Founder of The Unveiled Heart

TENACIOUS
grace

TENACIOUS
grace

Redefine Your Relationship
With Food and End Emotional Eating

JENNA BARBOSA

All Scripture quotations, unless otherwise indicated, are taken from the Holy Bible, New International Version®, NIV®. Copyright ©1973, 1978, 1984, 2011 by Biblica, Inc.™ Used by permission of Zondervan. All rights reserved worldwide. www.zondervan.com The "NIV" and "New International Version" are trademarks registered in the United States Patent and Trademark Office by Biblica, Inc.™

Scripture quotations marked (ESV) are from The ESV® Bible (The Holy Bible, English Standard Version®), copyright © 2001 by Crossway, a publishing ministry of Good News Publishers. Used by permission. All rights reserved.

Scripture quotations marked (NLT) are taken from the Holy Bible, New Living Translation, copyright ©1996, 2004, 2015 by Tyndale House Foundation. Used by permission of Tyndale House Publishers, Inc., Carol Stream, Illinois 60188. All rights reserved.

Scripture quotations taken from the New American Standard Bible® (NASB), copyright © 1960, 1962, 1963, 1968, 1971, 1972, 1973, 1975, 1977, 1995 by The Lockman Foundation. Used by permission. www.Lockman.org

Scripture quotations marked (CEV) are from the Contemporary English Version Copyright © 1991, 1992, 1995 by American Bible Society, Used by Permission.

The Holy Bible, Berean Study Bible (BSB), copyright ©2016, 2018 by Bible Hub. Used by Permission. All Rights Reserved Worldwide.

Scripture quotations marked HCSB®, are taken from the Holman Christian Standard Bible®, Copyright © 1999, 2000, 2002, 2003, 2009 by Holman Bible Publishers. Used by permission. HCSB® is a federally registered trademark of Holman Bible Publishers.

Printed in the United States of America
by Author Academy Elite
PO Box 43, Powell, OH 43065
www.AuthorAcademyElite.com

Paperback: ISBN 978-1-64085-963-0
Hardback: ISBN 978-1-64085-964-7
E-book: ISBN 978-1-64085-965-4

Library of Congress Control Number: 2019915299

Dedication

This book is for you — *you*, who feels caught in the cycle of either loving or fearing food just a little too much and then disliking yourself because of those emotions.

You, who feels your identity is wrapped up in how your body looks or feels.

You, whose body exposes your secret relationship with food.

You, who desires to please God with the body He has given you but don't know how to do that on a daily basis.

You, who has been diagnosed with an eating disorder and struggles to believe you are not your disorder.

You, who has tried countless "how-to" programs and diets to fix your insatiable hunger for or fear of food only to feel them increased.

This book is for you — and me. God has freedom for us. It's our time. He will have compassion on us. He longs to be gracious to us — and that grace is so tenacious.

Table of Contents

Foreword

A few months after I met Jenna at a speaking event, she asked if I would read the book she was getting ready to publish.

Knowing how much she had impacted women through her Christian counseling and support groups, I was so excited to have the chance to learn more about her story and how she helps women struggling with emotional eating—a topic I know all about. I struggled with closet binge eating from the age of 13 to 32, an addiction that eventually morphed into a 10-year drinking addiction.

Right as I started reading the introduction and saw the line "you have been trying to give *how* answers to a *why* question," I knew that this book could have completely changed my life had I read it when I was younger. Or anytime, actually. No one had ever explained my connection to food the way she did.

Not only would it have opened my eyes to the pain I was trying to ignore and hide with food, but it also would have helped me see that I was using food to numb and forget deep wounds that could only be healed by God.

It's amazing how much we can't see when we are so consumed with shame and guilt.

Food was my drug of choice. I tried to quit my binging thousands of times, but I was obsessed with when I could get my next fix.

I continued to run to food for emotional comfort even though it left me feeling empty and hopeless. Because I didn't understand my relationship with food and why I binged, I would simply exchange that drug of choice for alcohol and continue to numb the pain for many more years.

I believe that our stories are some of the most powerful ways God can use us to help others overcome their struggles. And that's what Jenna is doing with this book—helping people overcome lifelong battles. Jenna's gift to us is her story. She's giving us the opportunity to discover our pain and see our emotional eating in a completely different way. She's helping us find comfort in knowing that we are not alone.

We no longer need to hide in shame and pull away from God. Instead, we can seek God, knowing that He can break us free from what seems like a toxic, abusive relationship.

Tenacious Grace is an invitation to see emotional eating through the eyes of God so that we can learn to satisfy our spiritual hunger with His unconditional love. We can finally break out of the isolation and shame and find true joy.

—Virginia Kerr

Former TV news anchor and current CEO of This Is Virginia Kerr — video marketing and branding consultation for small business owners.

Acknowledgments

This book and the healing God did in me through not only writing it but living it out were God's answers to my prayer and I have so many to thank, but here are some special mentions.

First and foremost, I thank God, who is our Great Healer. He led me out to the wilderness with loving hands to heal the broken places within me, to teach me His truths over Satan's lies, and to provide resilience and strength for the many trials along the way. In all these, God has been and continues to be so faithful to me. Because He desires wholeness in us, He didn't only heal my idolatrous relationship with food, but He also healed my codependency with men. I am so glad I've chosen time and time again to remain walking under His loving arms, even in a wilderness, so that I can now walk in His promises of freedom in a new way.

To all of you who were part of the first four pilot support groups—thank you! Your trust in me to lead you on a journey that I was walking myself will never be forgotten. The vulnerability you all showed allowed everyone who participated to reach new levels of freedom. There is such beauty in standing together and working through the hard stuff, regardless of where we are in our own healing journeys. Thank you for being the chalkboards on which I was able to dream with God and practice how the future of Tenacious Grace Support Groups would look and how they could best help those who participate. I will forever cherish the memories we made together.

To all of you who have hired me as your Tenacious Grace Coach—thank you! For you to invest financially in our one-on-one journey and to allow God to use me in the deeper places of your heart and life means so much. The work you put in inspired me to continue putting the emotional effort into my own journey. I am excited about the future of Tenacious Grace Coaching and how it will impact the lives not only of those who seek out coaching but those who become certified coaches themselves.

This book could not have been a success without the support of my inner-circle people: those who held space for my vulnerability and struggles, pointed me to Christ, and cheered me on. To my family—Daddy, Momma, Anna, Chez, and Charity—thank you so much! God has used you all to make me who I am today. From the hard conflicts to the love, loyalty, and laughter, I am so grateful for it all. Your support and prayers mean the world to me. Luke, thank you for your support, love, and friendship from so very early on in your relationship with Anna. You have played a part in helping me continue my journey of waiting for God's best in my life. I'm excited to call you brother-in-law! I've been blessed with having a front-row seat to watch God's grace work in some incredible ways within our family. I love each of you dearly.

To my sisters in Christ who have been up close and personal to my ups and downs along this freedom journey—our many shared prayers and conversations have given me the courage to stay on the operating table as God does surgery on my heart regarding so many issues beyond my food struggles. Bess, Angie, Chrissy, Christina, Elizabeth, and Dionne, thank you so much for your love, prayers, support, friendship, and accountability. For speaking the truth in love and lifting my head to look at Jesus, I will forever be grateful for you and so blessed by you.

I want to thank my dear sisters and brothers in Christ who are in and connected to some powerful ministries—Christy and the ladies of Fearless Women and Jayne and the ladies of Altered Ministries. Thank you, Carrie G., for listening to God's leading and joining the team at such an early stage. Thank you, Megan, Roxanne, Greg, Matt, Micah, and my NorthRoad church family who have prayed for, asked about, and welcomed me as one of your own.

Virginia, thank you for trusting me and this message enough to write the foreword to this book for my readers. I know your experiences, vulnerability, and love for God and people will impact so many lives.

Megan, thank you for your friendship and your creative design work for the chapter about shame. I know it will help my readers better understand how shame effects their lives as they remember your great visual illustration. Your talent and art with Newberry Squared will impact so many.

Thank you to my counselor, MaryAnne, for tending to my heart and emotional ups and downs as I learned to stand firm on God's truths that overrode such deep-seated faulty belief systems. God used you mightily to help me build the spiritual and emotional muscles needed to birth the elephant of a baby that is this book and what is to follow.

To my personal trainer, Stacie, who for years now has provided friendship and accountability that has kept me committed to taking care of *me*—even in the face of hard times in life. Your ability to adjust your level of support to the exhausting years of being on my roller coaster of relational, emotional, and physical ups and downs has been so valuable to me. I have loved the fact that you knew some days I needed lighter workouts accompanied by more emotional support while other days you knew I needed to put the heavy workout in to push through the emotional stuff. Thank you, friend.

To my Facebook family—you all have been cheerleaders, prayer warriors, and friends. Thank you for following what God is doing in my life and along this journey. You provide a large part of my platform to share God's truth and accomplish my mission of inspiring resilience while leading you to the heart of Jesus.

Introduction

Are you fed up with trying to understand your struggle with food? Is it on your mind more often than you would like? Maybe food isn't merely food to you. Perhaps you run to it for relief or run from it out of guilt and fear. You've recognized that food has power over your emotions, and you feel frustrated and helpless.

If you are reading this book, you may be at a place of realization. You have been trying to give *how* answers to a *why* question. You're realizing the math doesn't add up. You follow the program for a while until you don't. Why? You stay in the gym for a while until you don't. Why?

I'm with you. I've asked the same question so many times. I've made countless lists of what I'll do differently with a resolve to overcome while also crying so many tears from feeling powerless in this struggle. When it really comes down to it, we don't know how to answer that *why* question. We say, "I'm too busy," or, "I don't have the willpower," but the more we hear ourselves justify our failure to stay on track in getting healthier, losing weight, and overcoming the power food has over us (yet again), the more frustrated we become. We give up for a while until the struggle becomes too loud, and then we're back on the same well-worn track: the same diets, programs, groups, trips to the grocery store, time reading through recipes, Pinterest ideas, and so many more how-to tips and tricks. The cycle continues. Some of us may lose weight and feel great—until something stressful puts us right back on the scales and in the stores to buy new clothes for our expanding waistline.

I have found that there are people who *overeat* and then there are people who *emotionally* eat. There's a big difference. People who view food as fuel do well with managing their intake. When they overeat, they feel physical discomfort. Rather than experiencing feelings of guilt, they regret eating too much. They finally get to a point where they realize they aren't taking care of their body the way they know they should. These feelings of regret lead them to put a plan in place to lose weight, and they stick with it. Those who don't have emotional tethers to food don't have the same struggle with food and emotional eating. Their battles look different. This isn't their story.

This is the story of the other type of people—people like you and me who attach feelings to food. Some eat not only to enjoy the taste but also to make their hearts taste something. Others restrict eating for fear of how gaining weight will impact them.

Food means something to all of us. To people who do not attach emotionally to food, it is their fuel. To those of us who struggle with emotional eating, it's our protection, escape, love, friendship, companionship, success, control, and much more. The meanings are endless when we believe that food can be anything more than what it was created to be: fuel.

We can't identify the source of our emotional eating until we stop long enough to put our eyes on the deeper issue. Emotional eating begins in different ways; we all have a unique story. Some, like me, have struggled since childhood due to a traumatic experience. For others, the problem arose after a sports injury knocked their career off track. Some didn't have an issue with emotional eating until they had their babies. The causes vary, but the result is the same. We eat not to fuel our bodies but to fix our emotions. The fulfillment we believe food provides starts to crumble after we realize it never lasts long—it's just a temporary patch.

I have struggled with emotional eating since I was a child. After going through a traumatic experience of being sexually molested at eight years old, food became my escape. I felt that food "approved" of me in the midst of feeling so much rejection from my abuser. It gave me a concrete place for my very confused and shameful thoughts to land. Food offered me an external sense of control to cover my internal feeling of insecurity.

My identity and worth had been hijacked, and the trauma laid a foundational — yet extremely faulty — belief system. I wrongly believed that getting approval from someone meant going along with everything they wanted. As a teenager, I felt completely insecure on the inside while acting secure on the outside. I felt my voice fade into the background when it came to things I wanted in life and relationships — also fading was my power to say no.

This feeling of powerlessness that can come with sexual abuse and trauma was reinforced every time I felt food call my name. It was reminding me I could escape into it from that internal storm. For example, at youth events where I felt awkward and insecure (desperately trying to fit in), the pizza on the buffet table was a welcome distraction. It rescued me from the uncomfortable feeling of being out of place. Everyone was eating the pizza, so I was included. Every slice solidified the belief I wasn't alone and by some chance could be approved of as a peer — as long as I had the food.

Food moved into my mind and set up camp early on, whether I liked it or not.

This pattern of running to food carried into my young adulthood. When I saw friends and family move on in life, get married, and have kids, food was my emotional support. When I was in an extremely lonely and emotionally abusive relationship, food was my companion in the loneliness. Pizza was either picked up or delivered too many times to count. My dependence on food started from one event but was reinforced by other events.

I was exhausted by the constant battle. I couldn't be at a party without having my internal compass point to where the food was. I couldn't have a small amount of food without thinking I could grab more when I got home. I couldn't be at a restaurant and choose not to eat if I wasn't physically hungry.

This battle led to excess weight gain—external evidence of my internal fight. I was on the losing side. Invitations to camp, swim, hike, travel, or take part in other fun athletic adventures would always trigger thoughts of how I would hold up physically. Fear of what others would think plagued my thoughts so much that I made jokes about me being "fluffy" in an attempt to beat them to the punchline. Maybe if I seemed to be OK with my size, they wouldn't think I was "less than."

The psychological term to define this type of self-protection is impression management. I was always attempting to manage or influence people's impression of me by being extra friendly, funny, cute, and helpful. On the flip side, I would manage their impressions of me by not being around them (isolation and avoidance).

I can't begin to convey on paper the emotional exhaustion I felt inside. After 22 years of this, I'd had enough.

I cried out to God and asked Him to reveal to me what was in my heart and mind that kept me prisoner to food. "Why can't I overcome this addiction to food? It shouldn't be this hard. Food is just food, isn't it?" I needed an answer that focused on emotional eating, not the typical "follow a new diet" advice. I realized I couldn't answer *why* questions with *how* answers anymore.

I asked God to teach me, heal what was broken within me, and guide me to freedom. He answered my questions. I couldn't overcome this struggle with food because I wasn't viewing it the way God did. He had to show me His perspective: Food wasn't fuel to me—it was my "fix."

Feeling a bit discouraged at these new revelations, I remembered that doing it my way had failed miserably. I was ready (as ready as I could be) to have God teach me something new. Little did I know that He wanted to use *me* to teach *you*.

God reminded me that He wants my freedom from emotional eating. He wants my allegiance and my whole heart. I'm not the only one who wants us to walk in freedom — God sent His son, Jesus, to die for this very reason: to set the captives free. Jesus wants you to walk in freedom from emotional eating. God wants your allegiance and your whole heart. He promises you will find Him when you seek Him with all your heart.

In Galatians 5:1, Paul writes, "It is for freedom that Christ has set us free. Stand firm, then, and do not let yourselves be burdened again by a yoke of slavery." A yoke in this verse refers to a heavy burden, comparable to the heavy yokes that are placed around the necks of oxen or bulls to carry a load. When we accept Christ as our Savior and begin that relationship with Him, we are set free from the bondage of sin.

Often though, we choose to stay in the prison of that sin we have been freed from. It's like a prisoner who has been released returning to their cell. We continue to put ourselves under the heavy weight of our belief system that emotional eating is the place to seek shelter instead of Jesus. This is what is called a spiritual stronghold.

It's time to walk in the freedom that Jesus died for. It's time to step out of the cell and off the prison grounds. God revealed to me that the name of this journey is "Tenacious Grace."

When we look at the definitions of *tenacious*, we see that it means "tending to keep a firm hold of something; clinging or adhering closely."[1] God is tenacious in His desire for and pursuit of our hearts. He is tenacious in His intention to be our complete fulfillment because He is the only One who can fulfill our hearts.

Grace, when used as a noun, means having good will toward someone; it's a condition or fact of being favored.[2] God's heart is *for* us, not against us! His favor is freely given as a blessing to us. It is not earned by our performance. No matter what we do or don't do, we have always been, we are, and we will always be favored by God. Yes, there are consequences to sin, but our status of approval and good standing with God does not change.

When grace is used as a verb, it means to do honor or credit to someone by one's presence.[3] Jesus graced us with

His presence when He walked on this earth as a man so that, through His death and resurrection, He could provide salvation to us sinners. He didn't stop there — once we accept the gift of salvation, we are graced with the presence of His Holy Spirit who dwells within us. The Holy Spirit empowers us to walk this journey and live in freedom.

When God showed me the curriculum for this journey, I felt as though I couldn't keep up, He was revealing it so quickly. I needed support and wanted to get the information God was giving me into the hands of women in my life who also needed help. Thus the Tenacious Grace Support Groups were born. These groups provide a place of understanding and exploration, uncovering why we emotionally eat or restrict food. If you are not part of a group, I encourage you to get connected with one. Information about these can be found in the back of this book.

From those first pilot groups came this book. For you. Whether or not you are in a group, this book will lay out a journey for you to uncover the deeper sources of your struggle. You will learn what God says about emotional eating and build a toolkit of truths, new revelations, and practical steps to help you win the war. This toolkit will be tailored to your personality, lifestyle, and relationship with God.

We who struggle with food tend to beat ourselves up and pull away from God in the areas that caused us to reach for food in the first place. We distance ourselves from Him instead of pressing into Him more closely. As we learn more about God's tenacious pursuit of our hearts and the freedom He has for us through His grace, we will peel back the layers of understanding the *why* behind our emotional eating.

As we embark on this journey, I'll be the first to say this looks like a daunting uphill climb. But take heart, my friend! God promises us a lot in Isaiah 45:1–6 (New Living Translation):

> This is what the Lord says to Cyrus, his anointed one, whose right hand He will empower. Before him, mighty kings will be paralyzed with fear. Their fortress gates will be opened, never to shut again. This is what the Lord says:

"I will go before you, Cyrus, and level the mountains. I will smash down gates of bronze and cut through bars of iron. And I will give you treasures hidden in the darkness — secret riches. I will do this so you may know that I am the Lord, the God of Israel, the one who calls you by name.

"And why have I called you for this work? Why did I call you by name when you did not know me? It is for the sake of Jacob my servant, Israel my chosen one. I am the Lord; there is no other God. I have equipped you for battle, though you don't even know me, so all the world from east to west will know there is no other God. I am the Lord, and there is no other."

There are a few things I want to highlight from this passage. First, Cyrus was a Persian king who didn't know or worship God. God chose him for a particular purpose. God's purpose was to show His people that in comparison to the many pagan idols of that time, God was the only One to be served. He was the only One who could fulfill what their hearts were looking for.

If God could take someone who didn't serve Him and lead him victoriously in battle, how much more will He lead you into victory? Cyrus was an instrument in God's hands to restore His people after their exile. God can use anyone to bring about His purpose, no matter how much they have blown it and feel far from God, He will still restore them.

God leads us to victory by empowering us. We must surrender to what He is doing. Cyrus yielded to what God wanted to do in using him for the restoration of Jerusalem. We must continually yield to God's strength throughout this journey.

I love the part where God says He will go before Cyrus and level the mountains. What is your mountain? Is it excess weight, old habits, trauma, a mindset, or your circumstances? Remember, this battle is one that will be won by following God as He goes before you and levels this mountain.

God also tells Cyrus that he will receive hidden treasures along the way. There are truths not yet revealed to you because you haven't walked this journey yet. God will reveal these hidden things and use them to restore you and lead you to victory.

His love convinces us that if we confess our sins, He is faithful to forgive them (1 John 1:9). He calls us deeper and whispers that He has so much more for us than sin can offer. Our core verse for this journey says it all:

> Therefore the LORD longs to be gracious to you,
> And therefore He waits on high to have compassion on you.
> For the LORD is a God of justice;
> How blessed are all those who long for Him.
> —Isaiah 30:18 (New American Standard Bible)

The context of this verse is God speaking to Israel when they were in rebellion, not when they had it all together! He is speaking this to us now, in our time of need.

God is tenacious in His pursuit of your heart. He longs to show you that He is the One who calls and equips you, empowers and sustains you, rewards and fulfills you. He will bless you and has called you by name.

Here we go.

PART ONE:

Redefine Your Relationship With Food

CHAPTER 1

"Hi there, this is food. We need to talk."

There I was, sitting in the front seat of his blue pickup truck with the lingering question, "What kind of relationship is this?" We'd started as friends, but it was growing into something more for me. It seemed as though it was for him too. It was time for the Talk.

When I was a freshman in college, this handsome guy sat behind me in class. Matt was an amazing guy, and as our classes progressed, so too did our friendship. He would pick me up late at night to get ice cream while we studied. We had many conversations about all things college and life. We began to go to church together, and I even hung out with his family. During homecoming festivities, the college held a bonfire after the coronations of the homecoming court. I was crowned freshman class homecoming princess that year, and as I was walking over to the bonfire, there was Matt—running over to me with excitement in his eyes. I felt my heart skip a beat as I saw him approaching me with the glow of the fire behind him.

3

When I felt his sweet hug, that was the moment I realized I had feelings for him beyond friendship.

I didn't fully realize my feelings had grown so much until our friendship failed to turn into the relationship I wanted in the timeframe I expected it to. After that night at the bonfire, I expected things to quickly and naturally fall into place for a romantic relationship. I began wanting our friendship to meet deeper needs and desires within my heart. In a small Christian university where the ongoing themes were "ring before spring" and "get your Mrs. Degree," I had unknowingly wrapped up my identity and worth in finding my soulmate and heading toward marriage.

After six months, Matt *still* wasn't asking me to move to the next step in our relationship, but I clearly saw that he liked me as more than a friend. I grew increasingly frustrated at the mixed messages.

When a friendship starts turning into something different, it's time for the awkward DTR (defining the relationship) Talk. This is important for both parties to know where the relationship stands and to avoid any hurt feelings due to misunderstood intentions. If we don't take the time to identify what is happening within a relationship, then we leave plenty of potential for pain.

Have you ever stopped long enough to define your relationship with food? First, you need to find out whether you and food are in an emotional relationship. This requires being honest with yourself and looking at how you interact with food. Because so many of us feel confused or uncomfortable about our relationship with food, we tend to look beyond the reality of our situation. An example of this is when jeans no longer fit — we wear yoga pants all the time instead of stepping back and looking at the deeper reasons behind our wardrobe shrinkage.

Ask yourself if you eat to live or live to eat. Some of you may eat whatever you want whenever you want it, regardless of what it does to your body. Others may do the opposite, eating very little or nothing at all as a way of attempting to stay in control.

When we get honest with ourselves, we can admit that we have been more tenacious in attempting to satisfy the cravings of our hearts with food than in seeking God for that fulfillment. We are in a full-blown emotional relationship with food, yet we deny the havoc it's wreaking in our hearts.

Denying this emotional relationship with food while trying to deal with the physical, spiritual, and emotional consequences of it in our daily lives is like trying to complete a jigsaw puzzle without looking at it. Take a few minutes and try putting a puzzle together with your eyes closed. It's impossible. That small amount of aggravation pales in comparison to the frustration of dealing with our emotional issues with food. Without looking directly at our relationship with food, we can't expect to put the pieces together.

> Denying this emotional relationship with food while trying to deal with the physical, spiritual, and emotional consequences of it in our daily lives is like trying to complete a jigsaw puzzle without looking at it.

Speaking of frustration, there I was—sitting in the front seat of Matt's truck defining the relationship. I got my answer. I was walking a path toward romantic love faster than he was. Along that path, my actions toward him had started to change. I was viewing him differently than a college friend, and I'd placed unrealistic expectations on him that weren't yet his to meet. After that DTR, everything changed. Once I intentionally redefined how I interacted with him due to my new awareness about our relationship, we no longer had emotional ties. He went his way and I went mine.

Wherever you are today, this is your front seat moment. It's time for your DTR with food.

If I asked you to introduce me to a family member or a friend, you would at least tell me two identifying factors: their name and their relationship to you. I'd like for you to introduce me to your food. Name it and its relationship to you. What is food, in general, to you? What do specific foods mean to you? We often find out what they mean to us by asking how we felt before eating them. When we do this enough, we can see certain foods attached to specific feelings. These feelings can stem from situations that laid faulty belief systems in our hearts.

Let me share an example introduction from my own journey: "This is my companion when I'm lonely, and its name is pizza. Our relationship started when I was a youth and felt insecure at group events. When everyone ate pizza together, I felt included and not as lonely and insecure. This was reinforced when, as an adult, I was in a toxic relationship with a man for seven years. I would turn to pizza for comfort in my deep loneliness."

It's your turn. Grab your journal or a piece of paper and get honest with yourself. Write down your go-to foods on one column and the emotional attachment you have with them on the other. Here is an example to get you started:

My Go-To Foods:	I Feel This Way Before Choosing That Food:
Pizza	Lonely
Fast food	Overwhelmed

Don't get stuck here. Don't overthink this. I didn't make these connections right away but rather as a result of continually observing my own actions, thoughts, and feelings.

For those of you whose emotional relationship with food centers around restriction, there is a little different approach to identifying your relationship with food. The major underlying emotion with the restrictive type of emotional eating is fear. The key is to determine which fears attach to the foods you avoid or that cause you anxiety when thinking about them. Ask yourself which experiences you avoid because food will be present, which specific foods you restrict, and lastly, identify the specific fears or thoughts driving your choice to restrict.

Experiences:	Foods I Restrict or That Cause Me Anxiety:	I'm Afraid This Will Happen If I Eat the Food:
Restaurants	Fried Foods	People will see me eating "bad" food.
It doesn't matter	High-calorie foods	I'm afraid I'll get fat.

FINDING GROUND ZERO

We've established that you have an emotional relationship with food. Next, we must determine if this relationship is a result of an altered state of perception. This means you believe food has the capability to interact with you on a heart level. This, my friend, is your ground zero—the starting point from which you will forge a new connection with food.

Now we can begin to unpack the many different aspects of our relationship with food and begin to identify our *why*. As we answer this *why* behind our emotional relationship with food, it is all too easy to jump headfirst into a specific diet plan or program. Instead, you need to pause and remind yourself that yet another "how-to" will not answer your *why* question.

There are so many diet plans out there, and each of them has its own research and ideas on how its way is the best way to eat and get healthy. Unfortunately, the majority of these methods target the physical changes and overlook the triggers and reasons why there is an issue to begin with. The emotional catalysts that lead to the physical results of being over or underweight (along with a variety of other health struggles) are overlooked by most health plans.

The harsh reality is that if merely knowing *how* to change our physical weight and health issues were all it took to overcome emotional eating, none of us would struggle with it. For years I knew how to change my weight, but I realized it didn't work long-term because I always gained it back, and eventually

I couldn't even get going on any new program long enough to see results.

Paul tells us not to let the differing opinions of what to eat or not eat distract us from relationships with one another. In 1 Corinthians 10:23–31 (NLT), Paul addresses the issue of how serving food sacrificed to idols can bring up an argument about whether or not that food is OK to eat. This is not far removed from the diet culture of today where people are arguing about which diet is best.

> You say, "I am allowed to do anything" — but not everything is good for you. You say, "I am allowed to do anything" — but not everything is beneficial. Don't be concerned for your own good but for the good of others.
>
> So you may eat any meat that is sold in the marketplace without raising questions of conscience. For "the earth is the Lord's, and everything in it."
>
> If someone who isn't a believer asks you home for dinner, accept the invitation if you want to. Eat whatever is offered to you without raising questions of conscience. (But suppose someone tells you, "This meat was offered to an idol." Don't eat it, out of consideration for the conscience of the one who told you. It might not be a matter of conscience for you, but it is for the other person.) For why should my freedom be limited by what someone else thinks? If I can thank God for the food and enjoy it, why should I be condemned for eating it?
>
> So whether you eat or drink, or whatever you do, do it all for the glory of God.

What Paul is saying here is that the heart connection with people (for the hope of bringing them closer to Christ) is more important than the food on the table. He puts food in its place: food is food. There are so many different diets out on the market, and each one has something to say about the others. People are divided by arguments over which way of eating is the best. The issue isn't to focus on convincing others to eat our specific way but instead to focus on building relationships and paying attention to the position of our hearts.

Paul was trying to teach that we are free to eat anything — but before we do, we must use wisdom. Because we connect emotions with food so often, it becomes more of an issue than it needs to be in our daily lives.

Paul also tells us that food is going to fuel the body but never satisfy the heart. He gives the meal and eating a spiritual focus — where the heart is — instead of placing the focus on the food. We have the freedom to eat all foods, but is it wise to do so? We need to approach eating with a standard of godliness. Every body is different, and we alter our God-made bodies into self-remade bodies by the foods we put in them. Once we stop eating emotionally and start choosing foods that fuel our bodies, our remade bodies will naturally become healthier. From here — ground zero — we begin to build.

COMFORT, THY NAME IS CHOCOLATE

Food was given to us as fuel for our bodies — not as a fix for our emotions. However, this doesn't mean we can't enjoy the taste of food. God blessed us with taste buds so we can enjoy the taste of food as it nourishes our bodies. God enjoys detail and embellishment. Just look at all the fun and beautiful designs of flowers, birds, plants, snowflakes, trees, people, and so many more intricacies in nature. God enjoys His own creation and wants us to enjoy it as well, but it was never intended to be worshipped. A healthy relationship with food is one that views food as fuel for our bodies that just happens to taste wonderful. An emotional relationship with food views it as having the ability to fix or fulfill something within our hearts.

Both positive and negative emotions can intertwine our heartstrings with food. When we believe that celebrating anything means there must be a social event around a meal, there's a positive association between celebration and food. It goes off-track when we find ourselves unable to enjoy an event without eating, even if we aren't hungry physically. We have just turned a positive emotion into a negative emotional relationship with food.

In elementary school, I learned about personification: attributing human characteristics to something nonhuman.[4] I remember drawing a picture of the sun with a smiling face in it. I then wrote "the sun smiled at me" on my paper. Obviously, the sun cannot smile since it doesn't have a mouth, but you can almost imagine a beam of sunlight as a warm smile.

We often personify food. The term "comfort food" demonstrates this clearly. We believe food will comfort, protect, validate, affirm, cause us to feel loved, or be our companion. We say things like "I'll get my hugs from food," "Ice cream is my friend," and "I'll eat my feelings" all in an attempt to redirect what may be stirring emotionally under the surface.

Believing that food can bring emotional fulfillment to our hearts is like walking through the day wearing a virtual reality headset. It creates an altered state of perception. Until we take off the headset and look through the lens of reality, we cannot break free. I'm not saying we're completely out of touch with reality, but when it comes to our belief system, we are deceived if we think that food can fix emotional wounds or serve as a replacement for our heart's desires.

When talking about emotional eating, I tend to use a car as a metaphor. A car needs fuel to run and get to its destination. Similarly, our bodies need fuel to function and get to our destinations in life. If I pulled my car up to a water hose and filled the tank with water, believing it would make my car run, you would look at me as if I'd lost my marbles. Not only would I go nowhere, but it would also do serious damage to my engine.

When we have an emotional relationship with food and turn to that to meet our needs, it's the same as driving our cars up to a water hose. We get nowhere near freedom, and it does serious damage to our emotions, bodies, and relationships. How can we be ready to go and do anything for God to the best of our ability when our ability is limited by an unhealthy body and mind due to emotional eating issues? Thankfully, this damage is reversible through the power of Jesus that brings us to victory through this journey.

Now that we have made a determination about your relationship with food, we'll need to begin calling it what it is and keep our eyes on the puzzle pieces as we move forward. This process can be tricky and, at times, overwhelming. I want to encourage you to keep moving forward and to know that it will all eventually click into place.

GOING DEEPER

1. What's your story? How long have you been in an emotional relationship with food? Think back to when you first noticed changes in your eating behaviors, body image, desire for food, health issues, or weight gain. What was the root of those changes? Have you spent time figuring that out? What was happening in your life that pushed you into the "arms" of food?

2. How do you personify food? What human characteristics to you attribute to it? What positive and negative emotions have you attached to food, and where did those originate?

3. Do a damage assessment on your body, mind, emotions, and soul. How has emotional eating—like filling your gas tank with water—done damage and kept you from moving forward in life?

OWNING TRUTH

- I have a full-blown emotional relationship with food. The intensity of that relationship may look different for me than for others, but it is an emotional relationship.

- I will not be able to emotionally break up with food until I stop putting on the virtual reality headset and personifying food. Food cannot touch my heart in an emotional way. Food is food. Food is fuel.

- Like filling my gas tank with water, emotional eating is damaging me whether I admit it or not.

CHAPTER 2

Let's Just Call It What It Is

Walking along the streets of Matamoros, Mexico, I felt invigorated by the energy of the hustle and bustle of the marketplace. Tents and storefronts lined the cobblestone streets where locals and tourists shopped. I loved every part of it—the culture, the colors, the kaleidoscope of different foods and items to purchase.

I was seventeen years old and on a mission trip. The leaders told my group that the local merchants would expect us to negotiate prices with them. The merchants would start by trying to sell us their products at an inflated price. At first, haggling felt awkward, but after trying a few times, I began to feel confident. Each time I purchased a souvenir, I negotiated before exchanging the currency for it.

When we are triggered to eat emotionally, a negotiation process begins: we doubt God's truth and accept Satan's lies. This leads to the exchange of one belief system for another. This is how idolatry takes root. The longer we nurture the patterns of idolatry, the deeper those roots grow.

To identify something as idolatry, first, we must be clear on how God defines it. In Romans 1:25, Paul says, "They exchanged the truth about God for a lie, and worshipped and served created things rather than the Creator." An exchange always happens when we worship anything other than God.

Let's look at the negotiation process leading up to the exchange. What truths from God are we trading? What lies of Satan are we believing? The negotiation process is where we doubt God's truth that He can and will fulfill all our hearts' needs when we seek Him. We believe the lie from Satan that tells us food can and will fulfill all our hearts' needs and give us relief from the pain of our circumstances.

The currency we spend is our bodies, worth, and freedom. We walk away with a temporary emotional fix from food. When this transaction happens, we aren't giving God the chance to show His faithfulness and come through for us—and we continue the cycle of emotional eating.

As a single woman with no children, whenever I was triggered by yet another friend getting married or having a baby, I found myself negotiating my worth. I believed I was worth less than those friends receiving the blessings I desired. My unmet desires for those things increased my dependency on food.

My dissatisfaction made me doubt God's good plan for my life, and I exchanged the truth (*my relationship status doesn't determine my worth or identity*) for a lie (*because I'm not married and am left behind, yet again, I must not be worth a man's pursuit*). This negotiation process had me running to food to get an emotional fix for the pain. Every time I believed that lie, it chipped away at my worth. Believing I wasn't worth a man's pursuit led me to believe I wasn't worth my own effort to pursue a healthy relationship with food and my body—so the cycle continued.

The exchange of truth for lies can happen on many different levels. Stress could be a trigger that leads us to negotiate the truth that Christ brings peace for the lie that food can bring

14

peace. Perhaps social outings trigger the lie that socializing isn't as good if food isn't present.

Take a moment and journal the negotiations with Satan that you find yourself in.

IDOLS DON'T GIVE—THEY TAKE

As we found in the last chapter, we personify food and place emotional attachments on it that leave us feeling empty and frustrated. This lack of fulfillment is a burden we carry, and yet we keep going back to food, hoping that it will eventually meet our emotional needs. This is the definition of idolatry: a bottomless pit that can never satisfy.

I fell into the idolatry pit in my twenties.

I'd like to share a little more of my story with you — as if we were at a coffeehouse getting to know one another. My desire is that you don't compare your pain or your story to mine, but that you understand this core message: our biggest pain may be our biggest platform to launch us into the very freedom Christ obtained for us.

I've shared with you how I was sexually molested at eight years old. At that time, I couldn't emotionally process what was going on, so I disassociated emotionally from the reality of the situation and repressed the memory until I was twenty-one years old. During my teen years of battling against a growing dependency on food, Satan laid the groundwork for other lies that said I could be happier and more fulfilled if I had a husband, kids, good body, money, approval, control, popularity, and so much more. My identity was wrapped up in how well I could please others and gain their approval. This was all an attempt to secure those things I believed would bring me a deeper sense of satisfaction.

Another place I found a secure identity was in hiding in the shadow of my big brother. I often found comfort and happiness in having him around when going through hard things. Satan used my childhood pain and trauma to lay a faulty belief system that said my brother was my emotional safe place, my security.

This feeling of safety went beyond just big-brother protection. We were very close, and I unknowingly placed him in the most powerful place in my heart — giving him the power to fill the role of a savior and bring me emotional security.

I moved back home from college at twenty-one, shortly after my brother got married. The reality that my relationship with him was changing left me feeling like my emotional security had crumbled. I had learned to hide the real me who was insecure and fearful by making a large portion of our sibling relationship about him, his happiness, and keeping the focus on things in his life rather than mine. I believed that if I could help him be happy, then he wouldn't hurt me or leave me.

Then he left. He was still my brother who cared about me, and he didn't do anything other than move on with his new marriage and happiness. That was good for him, but I guess he never got the memo that he was supposed to stay on the throne of my heart as my savior. I laugh about that now because I want to go back to twenty-one-year-old Jenna and speak some solid truth to her. I would tell her that often when we give humans the God-sized task of being the source of our emotional security on an identity and worth level, we are deeply hurt by their actions when they do what's important and healthy for them. Things they do that we should celebrate instead hit a deep and unhealthy place in us that creates tension, bitterness, and distance.

This was the beginning of the necessary stripping away of my idols. Little did I know my brother was only the first one.

One day, the summer after moving home, while I was getting ready to go to the pool with my mom, sister-in-law, and sister, the memory of my sexual abuse at the age of eight came rushing back, full throttle. I felt as though all the pain of my teen years from food and relationships came crashing together.

After that, I had a hard time processing what had happened and began partying. I gave up my virginity (which I'd fiercely protected for years) because my identity and worth were not grounded in Christ. Remembering my traumatic experience was like a wrecking ball to the false sense of identity I had built around being my brother's little sister and a good Christian girl—I crumbled.

I quickly got into a relationship, and a few months later, I had a miscarriage. I was twenty-two years old, alone in my apartment, and barely able to process everything that had happened since I was a little girl—let alone the trauma of losing a baby. I collapsed. As I lay on my bathroom floor, I mourned the loss of what could have been. That seemed to be the theme of my pain: utter powerlessness and lack of control.

After that, I desperately tried to get my act together. I stayed sexually pure, I cleaned up my cussing, stopped drinking and partying, and stayed away from toxic people. I kept trying to clean up my behavior instead of asking God to reveal the state of my heart for the purpose of healing. I stayed in the mentality of cleaning myself up for two years.

Then I suffered another emotional blow to the heart with a different guy. I then plunged headfirst into this lie from Satan: *Waiting on God's timing and doing things His way doesn't bring happiness, so why not be your own god?* This turned into a belief system of full-blown idolatry that showed up in actions that revolved around toxic relationships, partying, self-protective coping methods like manipulation, and self-serving, unfiltered, and unfulfilling decisions made on impulse.

No one knew all the shame and pain I was carrying at that time. I felt alone, but at least I had food to comfort me. Or so I thought. In my attempts to find an emotionally strong footing, food was the number one thing I turned to when things got tough, yet it slowly betrayed me with every added pound and health issue that developed.

When we have exchanged God's truth for Satan's lie, time and circumstance lead us into doing things we never thought we would choose to do. I let my emotional pain run the show for close to seven more years. Idolatry is a pit, but we can decorate it in a way that makes us believe it's a comfort zone. Only

✖ Only when the pain of idolatry surpasses the pain of surrender do we begin to climb out of the pit.

17

when the pain of idolatry surpasses the pain of surrender do we begin to climb out of the pit.

The prophet Isaiah makes it clear that our idols are powerless to satisfy us by comparing God's actions to the inaction of false gods. Isaiah 46:7 (Contemporary English Version) says, "They carry the idol on their shoulders, then put it on a stand, but it cannot move. They call out to the idol when they are in trouble, but it doesn't answer, and it cannot help." Verses 5 and 6 (NASB) show us how God is the One who has the power to meet our needs: "Even to your old age I will be the same, and even to your graying years I will bear you! I have done it, and I will carry you; and I will bear you and I will deliver you. To whom would you liken Me and make Me equal and compare Me, that we would be alike?"

I tried for years to believe that food, sex, money, approval, and power were more powerful than God. These were the idols I worshipped. I carried their weight along with the emotional, physical, and spiritual consequences of my worship. Through that pain, I finally realized that no idol would ever deliver on the promise of lasting love and fulfillment that my heart longed for.

In the verses above, we can sense God's longing to be gracious to us. He clearly and repeatedly states that *He alone* can deliver on His promises—and He wants to.

Emotional eating is idolatry. Food is the idol we use to represent the god of selfish desire. We believe we have the power and knowledge to meet our own needs—and food is the way we do that. The truth is that only our Creator God has the power and knowledge to meet our needs—through Himself.

If you're anything like me, you've reached the point where you're exhausted from carrying the idol of food. You're tired of waiting for your emotional eating to come through for you and produce lasting results instead of more problems. You only feel emptier after every emotional binge or period of restriction.

Enough is enough. I've drawn a line in the sand and chosen to smash my idol of food and dethrone the god of selfish desire. I cling to Isaiah 46:5–6 and allow God to carry me and deliver me. Do I live that choice out to perfection? No. There are times I pick up a broken shard of that idol of food and selfishly believe it can offer me emotional comfort. Do I live that choice out to the best of my ability at the place I'm at in my journey? Yes. I keep moving forward and allowing God to prove His faithfulness to me.

Have you drawn a line in the sand yet? Have you resolved that no longer will you continue to carry the burden of your idolatry with food and the selfish desire to be your own god? If not, take some time and do so through prayer by asking God to do this through you. This is a process, so you still have work to do, but the real work won't start until you've made that internal decision to say "enough" and mean it.

IDOLATRY DISTORTS OUR REALITY

We believe that where we are is a "comfort zone" because we've gotten used to it. A comfort zone is "a place or situation where one feels safe or at ease and without stress."[5]

Let's look at the concept of comfort. You operate within two zones: emotional eating and biological eating. Ask yourself what's comfortable about the emotional eating zone. Eating whatever you want whenever you want can give a feeling of control.

What's uncomfortable is the unwanted pounds that pile on, diabetes, heart attacks, high blood pressure, heartburn, digestive issues, fertility issues, broken relationships, the consequences of the sin of idolatry, guilt, shame, low self-esteem, distorted body image, clothes that don't fit . . . the list goes on. However, it's easy to feel that this zone is comfortable because it's familiar. When we adjust to uncomfortable consequences instead of changing the cause of those consequences, we live with an autopilot mentality.

Colossians 3:5 (English Standard Version) says, "Put to death therefore what is earthly in you: sexual immorality, impurity, passion, evil desire, and covetousness, which is idolatry." Some of us may struggle with other things on this list, but let's focus on passion. This word passion is used to denote an "inordinate affection or lust."[6] How many of us can confirm that when we want that food fix or need to abstain from food, we can get quite passionate about it? That passion may manifest itself differently in different people, but none of us feel settled until we exert our control in getting what we want. We have an inordinate affection for food as our source of control.

This, my friend, is what is earthly in us—idolatry. When we engage in idolatry with one thing, we put out a welcome sign in neon lights for other types of idolatry. It's only a matter of time and circumstance before we are led into things we'd never thought possible. Our control within the emotional eating zone is a distorted view of control. In this zone, we end up being controlled rather than being the ones in control.

The second zone is our biological eating zone, which is where God wants us to stay. This zone can be comfortable because when we follow our bodies' signals and provide them with food as fuel, we have healthy working bodies. We are more active, our clothes fit better, our hormones are healthier, our mental clarity increases, and we are good stewards—or managers—of the bodies God has given us. When we honor God by presenting our bodies as living sacrifices, we have freedom, our self-esteem is higher, we spend less money on fast food, we have more confidence, and the list goes on.

The discomfort in this zone is that we must put to death our selfish desires and follow after Christ. We must set aside time for Bible study, plan meals, cook, make better choices about what we eat, exercise, and be intentional. Yes, these disciplines are uncomfortable, but as we continue to see the results that obedience brings, they will begin to feel more natural as we settle into a new lifestyle of freedom.

IDOLATRY IS DRIVEN BY PRIDE

In this exchange of God's truths for Satan's lies, we have put ourselves and food in a position of power above God. We are on the throne of our hearts, or "the God seat" as I like to call it. We follow our desires instead of God's commands. This is pride at its finest.

One way pride can show up with food is when we crave its taste more than we pay attention to its health benefits. When we're avoiding the uncomfortable aspects of changing, pride can lie to us and tell us it's not a big deal and we should do what feels good.

My mom would always tell us kids, "Don't rethink what I've told you. Just follow through with what I've already said." We rethink what God has told us. We negotiate with Satan. God tells us to put to death the earthly things within us, set our minds on things above, don't worship any other gods, and present ourselves as living sacrifices. Let's stop rethinking what God has told us.

Genesis 3:1–7 (NASB) says this:

> Now the serpent was more crafty than any beast of the field which the LORD God had made. And he said to the woman, "Indeed, has God said, 'You shall not eat from any tree of the garden'?" The woman said to the serpent, "From the fruit of the trees of the garden we may eat; but from the fruit of the tree which is in the middle of the garden, God has said, 'You shall not eat from it or touch it, or you will die.'" The serpent said to the woman, "You surely will not die! For God knows that in the day you eat from it your eyes will be opened, and you will be like God, knowing good and evil." When the woman saw that the tree was good for food, and that it was a delight to the eyes, and that the tree was desirable to make one wise, she took from its fruit and ate; and she gave also to her husband with her, and he ate. Then the eyes of both of them were opened, and they knew that they were naked; and they sewed fig leaves together and made themselves loin coverings.

Here we have the first case of emotional eating on record. Satan distorted Eve's thoughts, convincing her to act against God's protective design. He didn't start by directly contradicting

God's words; instead, he used a bit of truth to set a trap. He starts by repeating God's instructions, but he inserts one key word: *any*. In doing this, he caused Eve to doubt God's truth. Then he continued to flat-out lie to Eve about what God knew, and her eyes being opened, and she would be like God, blah blah, blah. His lies are always fluffed up with an ideal wish list. With this sleazeball strategy, he had Eve questioning God's faithful protection.

Could she be missing out on something? Was God holding out on her? Could she gain from a source other than God? Eve then personified the fruit, believing it to be capable of giving her wisdom, which she thought she lacked. She was walking with Wisdom Himself in the garden and was being protected from death under God's rule. Only after she believed Satan's lies and pridefully took control did she realize she had been duped.

COUNT THE COST

As with other idols, the idol of self requires sacrifices. We use food as the silver platter on which we serve up our self-worth, bodies, peace, and so much more. Every time we emotionally turn to food (a created thing), it costs us something.

What does it cost you? Money, health, relationships, self-esteem, bold decision-making? Spend some time and make a list of what your idolatry has cost you.

When we turn to God, it will also cost us something, but nothing compared to the high price of idolatry. The cost is surrender. We surrender our belief that we have the right to choose whatever we want whenever we want it.

In this journey of becoming more Christlike and overcoming idolatry, we must surrender to Jesus and take up our cross daily. Luke 9:22–24 (Berean Study Bible) says,

> "The Son of Man must suffer many things," He said. "He must be rejected by the elders, chief priests, and scribes, and He must be killed and on the third day be raised to life." Then Jesus said to all of them, "If anyone would come after Me, he

must deny himself and take up his cross daily and follow Me. For whoever wants to save his life will lose it, but whoever loses his life for My sake will save it."

At first glance, "coming after" Jesus looks uncomfortable. Taking up our cross doesn't seem too enticing, especially when the cross represents death. As born-again Christ followers, we have not only died—we have been raised to new life in Him! According to Colossians 3:1–4 (ESV), "If then you have been raised with Christ, seek the things that are above, where Christ is, seated at the right hand of God. Set your minds on things that are above, not on things that are on earth. For you have died, and your life is hidden with Christ in God. When Christ who is your life appears, then you also will appear with him in glory."

In everyday life, we tend to focus on our current pain and emotions instead of setting our minds on things above. When we are shortsighted and only focus on the temporary circumstances of life, we don't want our cross and aren't able to carry it. When we set our minds on things above and understand what "coming after" Jesus really means, we see what carrying our cross daily looks like. There are many blessings that come from persevering under the weight of our cross, and the most important one is *freedom*. Jesus persevered through every step of carrying His cross on the path toward the hill of Calvary. We were worth every single ounce of Jesus' steadfast resolve as He carried a cross to His own death.

What is our cross to carry when it comes to overcoming emotional eating? The answer is found in the finished work of the cross. We are to deny our selfish desire to meet our own needs and turn to food for an emotional fix. We are to intentionally carry the truth that we have access to everything we need to walk in freedom through the Holy Spirit within us. Thank God we were given the Holy Spirit of Jesus after His death on the cross and through His gift of salvation. He put to death our old self and made us a new creation through His blood. Therefore, we follow — we carry our cross daily — and God's grace is tenacious in helping us do just that.

IDOLATRY REINFORCES FAULTY RELATIONSHIP DEPENDENCY

"Taste and see that the LORD is good; blessed is the one who takes refuge in him" (Psalm 34:8). We are to "taste" and see that God is good. Instead, we "taste" food and create an unhealthy dependency on it. We put God-sized expectations on food, thinking it will meet our needs just as Eve thought the fruit would give her wisdom.

The personification of food started in the garden. The power of knowing good and evil wasn't in a fruit — it was in the disobedience to God's command. Eve's pride caused her to think she was on God's level and had the right to rethink what He had said. Her questioning God led to her act of disobedience. Then her husband, who was right there with her, passively stayed silent and ate the fruit as well. Like Eve and Adam, we focus too much on food and not enough on the position of our heart where pride and idolatry reside.

This dependency on food rather than God seeps into other areas of our lives. We can easily have a relational hunger for people, possessions, etc. that goes beyond what they are capable of providing. This hunger turns into a faulty belief system where we believe we *need* those things to have emotional security. We unrealistically expect created beings and things to have the capacity to hold the weight of our needs and in turn satisfy them better than our Creator. It's as if we're trying to fit a gallon of water into a Dixie cup. We cannot expect food, people, and things to meet our needs the way God can. If we do, we can become dependency-hoarders, grabbing onto anyone and anything that could potentially meet our needs.

Who or what else in your life are you "tasting" to see if it's good and able to meet your needs? The ability to discern what we are truly hungry for will help us continue walking in the right direction away from that line in the sand.

As I have intentionally fed my spiritual hunger, I've seen God work in so many amazing ways. The things and people I once grabbed onto for fulfillment have slowly been removed, and I've found freedom from toxic relationships and unhealthy thinking patterns. There has been an incredible increase in the peace my heart feels in the uncomfortable places within my wilderness walk.

GOING DEEPER

1. Every time we emotionally turn to food (a created thing), it costs us something. What does it cost you? Money, health, relationships, self-esteem, bold decision-making, something else?

2. What do you believe God is withholding from you that you can gain from emotionally eating?

3. When we are dependent on food to meet our emotional needs, we become dependency-hoarders. Who or what have you latched onto in a dependent way because of emotional eating?

OWNING TRUTH

- God defines idolatry as exchanging the truth about God for a lie, worshipping and serving created things rather than God, the Creator.

- In our idolatry of emotional eating, we put ourselves in "the God seat" and worship our selfish desire to eat what we want, when we want, and how much we want. We must get off the throne in our hearts and intentionally put God there instead.

- The power of knowing good and evil wasn't in a fruit — it was in the disobedience to God's command.

CHAPTER 3

Hungry Yet Never Satisfied

I love going to restaurants with people who try something new on the menu. I'm one of those people who will choose the same thing almost every time. I always look at the menu long and hard, trying to convince myself to choose something new. But ordering something different carries the risk of not liking it. That unknown means I inevitably pick what I'm familiar with because I know I'll enjoy it. If I'm lucky, I get to taste what my friends or family members order so I can try something new before I order it.

We can get stuck in our routines and choosing what we want when we want it simply because it's familiar. We give so much power to familiarity that we rarely step out of what we are used to. This can stem from good ole-fashioned selfishness.

We want to taste freedom without buying into it — committing to it. Many times, we have to be humbled by God and forced by circumstances to seek Him in the discomfort of freedom. Just as our tastes adjust to unfamiliar food over time, so will our desires and feelings adjust to the unfamiliarity of freedom. We must humble ourselves and allow God to teach us and help us walk confidently in the unknowns of a life of freedom from emotional eating. Let's do the humbling first before God has to do it for us.

> Just as our tastes adjust to unfamiliar food over time, so will our desires and feelings adjust to the unfamiliarity of freedom.

The Israelites were uncomfortable with the unfamiliarity of freedom. God's prescribed dose of humble pie for the pride in their hearts was 40 years in the wilderness. This was discipline for their idolatry, but it was rooted in love. He had brought them out of captivity, yet they were so focused on what they thought was the answer to their growing hunger—the familiar tastes and comforts they were used to in Egypt—that they began complaining and creating idols to worship instead of waiting on and trusting God. They were not committed to following Him into the unknowns of freedom, preferring to taste only its immediate feelings of release and excitement. Once that newness wore off and they felt uncomfortable, they wished they had stuck with their go-to comforts—even if that meant a life of captivity.

During their wilderness journey, they complained that manna (the food God provided for them) wasn't enough and they would rather go back to Egypt than continue eating it. My gut reaction to this is to think how crazy they were to desire the familiarity of captivity over the unknown of freedom simply because they were uncomfortable. Their focus was on their perceived lack of what they thought would be truly satisfying food. We, like the Israelites, often believe that our way with food can satisfy more than God's way. (Wisdom presents the question of how a created thing can be more satisfying than its creator.) We run back to being captive in this stronghold with food rather than remain uncomfortable in the wilderness times of freedom.

The reality was that the Israelites' physical hunger was being fully satisfied daily. The hunger they felt was spiritual.

Spiritual malnourishment will always cause emotional hunger. We then reach for food thinking it will satisfy and end up overfeeding the physical while starving the spiritual.

God loved them enough to reveal the *why* behind their idolatry, and in doing so, He revealed His power in being the true provider for their needs.

In Deuteronomy 8:1–5, Moses knows he will die before too long and gives some final leadership lessons to the people God used Him to lead out of slavery. He tells them,

> Be careful to follow every command I am giving you today, so that you may live and increase and may enter and possess the land the LORD promised on oath to your ancestors. Remember how the LORD your God led you all the way in the wilderness these forty years, to humble and test you in order to know what was in your heart, whether or not you would keep his commands. He humbled you, causing you to hunger and then feeding you with manna, which neither you nor your ancestors had known, to teach you that man does not live on bread alone but on every word that comes from the mouth of the LORD. Your clothes did not wear out and your feet did not swell during these forty years. Know then in your heart that as a man disciplines his son, so the LORD your God disciplines you.

The Lord has led us out into our wilderness to humble us and test us when it comes to keeping His commands. Our wilderness is this journey of God revealing the *why* behind our emotional eating and demonstrating that He is the true provider of our needs. He is teaching us to say no to the idols that kept us in bondage and yes to the one true God. He wants to show us that we can't live on bread alone, because we can eat all we want

Spiritual malnourishment will always cause emotional hunger. We then reach for food thinking it will satisfy and end up overfeeding the physical while starving the spiritual.

yet remain unsatisfied. We must live on God's words and cling to them so that we can walk in freedom.

Let's unpack three different types of hunger: emotional, physical, and spiritual. We all hunger for something, and depending on the day and circumstance, that hunger can easily change. The stronghold of emotional eating has funneled our hunger toward one answer: food. Instead of running straight to food, we need to shift our focus to identifying the type of hunger we're feeling and then choosing what will satisfy that hunger.

EMOTIONAL HUNGER

Emotion is defined as "a strong feeling deriving from one's circumstances, mood, or relationships with others." It is also defined as "instinctive or intuitive feeling as distinguished from reasoning or knowledge."[7] Emotions are not thoughts but are a result of thoughts based on circumstance, mood, or relationships. Emotions and feelings are synonymous, so I'll use the terms interchangeably.

If we follow our emotional hunger, we do what we feel instead of doing what we know to be true. The more we are led by feelings, the more our actions reinforce our false belief system. At the same time, emotions aren't bad, and they have their place. They are like toddlers. We can't let them drive our cars, but we can't stuff them in the trunk and ignore them either. We place toddlers in the back seat, buckled up securely, where we can keep an eye on them, engage with them, and protect them. We must do this with our emotions as well.

When we engage in emotional eating, our feelings are in the driver's seat. In that scenario, we crash and burn every time. It's important to highlight that *we* make this choice; no one else makes it for us. Our "choice button" is not broken. If we can choose to eat because of an emotional response, logically, we can choose *not* to eat.

There are many times when I have eaten a decent-sized meal and then immediately afterward told myself that I was still hungry. Other times, I would find myself saying "I'm hungry" out of the blue. It was automatic, as if my mind were on autopilot. In neither of those scenarios was I physically hungry. It wasn't until I went along this journey that I began to realize the patterns of those so-called hunger pains.

I noticed that I always felt "hungry" whenever I watched television. This would mainly happen with online streaming shows because all of the episodes were available—once I got hooked on the plot, it was so easy to let the next episode play automatically. Whenever I sat down to watch *Friends*, with its tight-knit group of characters, *Criminal Minds*, filled with suspense and excitement, or a romantic comedy (no matter how cheesy), I would get so wrapped up in what was happening that I felt a sense of loss after the series ended. I remember crying when my *Friends* marathon was over.

The lives of the people on the shows and movies were filled with excitement, romance, and intrigue, and it would trigger me to believe any number of colorful lies Satan chose to throw at me. The lies were mostly about how my life wasn't fulfilling because it didn't look like what I was seeing on those shows. I felt sad that I didn't have what brought those people happiness. Even though I knew these were fictional shows, the sadness still led me to believe I was lacking, that there was a void, and that food was the quick fix I needed.

Do you see the sly work of Satan's lies? Do you see how I exchanged the truth for a lie? Do you see the distorted reality of my reaction to a fictional show? These thoughts and feelings didn't happen within seconds. It was a slow, gradual process. The tipping point came when my emotions followed my thinking one minute too long, and that led me to emotionally eat.

I've been telling you how our emotions will lead our actions if we are in autopilot mode. You can see how those emotions are led by our thoughts. I was thinking about how my life wasn't as fulfilling as what I saw onscreen (thought), so I felt inferior (emotion), and this led me to pick up food (action). The action of eating ultimately reflected a core belief system. For a long time, I didn't realize it was my thinking that needed the fix, not my emotions.

Satan works like this. When we aren't being intentional with our mindsets — when we're on autopilot — he lays the bricks of a belief system that is held together by the mortar of his lies. These bricks make up walls that block our vision of what God is trying to show us. We must be more aware of the situations that trigger our wrong thinking so we do not act mindlessly out of emotional hunger.

PHYSICAL HUNGER

Eating is an essential part of keeping our bodies healthy, and our bodies are designed to give us cues when they need food. This leads me to one of the big differences between physical and emotional hunger: physical hunger has tangible — and sometimes even audible — effects. Physical hunger is defined as "a craving, desire, or urgent need for food. An uneasy sensation occasioned normally by the lack of food and resulting directly from stimulation of the sensory nerves of the stomach by the contraction and churning movement of the empty stomach."[8]

The problem is that if we're eating to satisfy our emotional hunger, we may never feel physical hunger. If we are continually eating, we don't give our bodies the chance to be physically hungry. How, then, can we recognize the prompts of physical hunger?

Everyone's hunger mechanism gives them different prompts. It's important to stop feeding emotional hunger long enough to get more in tune with the sensations of physical hunger. When I started focusing on my specific sensations, I learned that I get a burning feeling in my stomach that turns into an empty rumbling. At times, I can hear a growling sound. I also get slightly lightheaded and really tired.

The interesting thing is that when we become more aware of our bodies' physical cues, we see that in those moments of physical hunger we are not quite as passionate about eating as we are in emotional hunger moments. Eating becomes more of a to-do than a must-have. The more we make a choice to wait for that physical hunger sensation, the more we get to know our bodies and value them instead of hating them or feeling powerless within them. If we are operating out of physical hunger, we are free to choose what is best for our bodies.

Take a few moments and write down the specific sensations you're already aware your body uses as physical hunger signals. Then allow time for your body to get physically hungry and show you more.

SPIRITUAL HUNGER

The other kind of hunger pangs we feel indicate spiritual hunger. This can be defined as a sense of hopelessness and lack of satisfaction within one's soul, often following a focused perspective on surrounding circumstances. We see God's Word address spiritual hunger in Psalm 42:1–8.

> As the deer pants for streams of water,
> so my soul pants for you, my God.
> My soul thirsts for God, for the living God.
> When can I go and meet with God?
> My tears have been my food
> day and night,
> while people say to me all day long,
> "Where is your God?"
> These things I remember
> as I pour out my soul:
> how I used to go to the house of God
> under the protection of the Mighty One
> with shouts of joy and praise
> among the festive throng.
>
> Why, my soul, are you downcast?
> Why so disturbed within me?
> Put your hope in God,
> for I will yet praise him,
> my Savior and my God.

My soul is downcast within me;
therefore, I will remember you
from the land of the Jordan,
the heights of Hermon—from Mount Mizar.
Deep calls to deep
in the roar of your waterfalls;
all your waves and breakers
have swept over me.

By day the LORD directs his love,
at night his song is with me—
a prayer to the God of my life.

We see that the psalmist thirsted for God in the midst of emotional turmoil. This is a good reminder for us that our emotional struggles are often alarms that tell us we may be spiritually hungry. The psalmist remembers his time of "mountaintop" emotions and experiences with God and challenges his current emotions by asking the *why* question. He commands his very soul to put its hope in God. Faith is what pushes him to keep his eyes on God's protection and goodness. He recognizes there is spiritual hunger within his soul because he has allowed his circumstances to paint a picture of hopelessness.

The writer's food has been his tears and he has poured out his soul. In this time of yearning for life's circumstances to change, he remembers the closeness he once had with God and the peace that brought him. He compares it to his current situation where his feelings are controlling him and draws his own line in the sand. He commands his soul to shift its hope from circumstantial change to God, the Mighty One, his Savior.

Just like the psalmist, most of our emotional eating is a result of spiritual hunger. You may be saying, "But I spend time every day in the Bible." This is a great spiritual discipline that is necessary for walking in freedom. However, if you are not intentionally seeking God for the fulfillment and answers you are seeking in food, there is still a spiritual hunger that isn't being fed within you. God promises to be your fulfillment in

Psalm 107:9 where He says, "He satisfies the thirsty soul and fills the hungry soul with good things."

Above everything else I've done in my journey of overcoming emotional eating, seeking God to feed my spiritual hunger and letting Him fill my emotional needs has allowed me to walk in freedom. From this new dynamic, I've been able to interact with my physical hunger more often than not the way God designed—eating for fuel. The physical weight loss is happening as an external result of inward healing, but it's a slow process. I have to remind myself that the number on the scale doesn't determine my spiritual freedom. It's a great indicator to measure where I'm at in the journey, but I can't rely on it as proof of my freedom.

HMMM . . . WHAT TO EAT?

You know that moment—you're standing at the refrigerator door as your stomach yells at you to feed it, but you don't know what to eat. If you didn't take the time to prep some healthy options and your choices are a head of lettuce (that could turn into a salad if you made the effort) or a slice of pizza, you know which one you'll choose.

Now that we have learned to identify which type of hunger we're feeling, we need to be vigilant and prepared with healthy fuel. Go on a treasure hunt in God's Word and seek out different verses that will help you focus on how to feed the hunger once you've identified it. Here are some verses that can help you get started:

- **Emotional Hunger:** Follow Philippians 4:8 for help on what to think about while replacing Satan's lies. Read Matthew 6:33 for a reminder to seek what's truly important first and foremost.

- **Physical Hunger:** God shows us in Genesis 1:29 that "every seed-bearing plant on the face of the whole earth and every tree that has fruit with seed in it" will be food for us. Then He tells us in Genesis 9:3 that "everything that lives and moves about will be food for you. Just as I gave you the green plants, I now give you everything." It's important to note that wisdom is necessary to discern "everything." Food like donuts, pizza, and candy didn't exist in Adam and Eve's day. As we are walking in freedom from emotional eating, it's important to recognize that all our modern processed and sweetened foods most likely wouldn't be on God's good list. They are "permissible," but not necessarily beneficial (1 Corinthians 10:23). Without being legalistic, we can understand that some foods can create addictive responses and do damage to our bodies. This is especially true for the emotional eater.

- **Spiritual Hunger:** Follow Psalm 81:8–10 where God calls us to obedience, which is honoring our relationship with Christ. He asks us to praise and worship and remember His deliverance. He pleads with us to listen and not turn to other gods. He tells us if we will turn to Him, He will fill us. He promises us we will find Him when we seek Him with all our hearts.

Because God is a good Father who disciplines us to teach and set us free, He shows us that if we continue in our stubborn idolatry, we will feel the full, unfiltered weight of the consequences of our choices. This is shown in Psalm 81:11–16 when Israel did not listen and chose to turn to other gods. God gave them over to their stubborn hearts to follow their own plans. He reminded them that even their very food comes from the Lord, yet they stayed rebellious.

Friend, I have been at a place where God gave me over to my own heart, and it wasn't pretty. Remember when I told you I plunged deep into the pit of idolatry? This period of close to eight years is what my family and I refer to as "the great rebellion" or my "dark years." Using my pain as permission, I chose full-out rebellion against God and what I knew to be true.

36

After partying heavily for about six months, I met a man and got into a six-year relationship with him. We lived together, and I played wife and mother all while being my own god and doing as I saw fit to meet my own needs. As I lived out a version of myself I never want to meet again, God was allowing the consequences of my actions to put an enormous amount of pressure on my relationships with family, friends, myself, and — most importantly — Him. I never felt as alone and powerless to change things as when I was playing the role of god in my life. Following my own plans led to so much brokenness. My heart felt shredded time and time again by unrealized dreams and unmet desires and expectations I put on people and romantic relationships. The weight of the sin in my heart manifested as excess weight on my body, debt in my finances, toxic and unhealthy relationships, and continued sinful choices — all of which were results of idolatry, and it was all my own doing.

By the grace of God, I have learned the truth of Jeremiah 17:9 and Proverbs 4:23. The heart is deceitful, but we are to guard it because it is the wellspring of life. When we follow our own stubborn hearts that lead toward idolatry, God will allow what we follow after to be the very thing that breaks our stubborn hearts. When we follow God and place our hearts in His hands, we guard against idolatry and walk in freedom. There, we find a beautiful and deeply satisfying love relationship with Him.

Jeremiah 2:13 talks about what it looks like when we follow our hearts' desires instead of following God. "For my people have committed two evils: they have forsaken me, the fountain of living waters, and hewed out cisterns for themselves, broken cisterns that can hold no water." In ancient Israel, wherever rain was scarce, people would dig pits out of the limestone hillsides to hold water. They would line the cisterns with a sticky plaster to prevent the water from seeping out. Sometimes, a cistern's plaster lining would crack and all the water would drain out. Jeremiah used this analogy to explain how, like a broken cistern, people would turn to idol worship expecting it to quench their thirsty souls rather than turn to God as the Living Water and the true source of sustenance for their souls.

We can apply what God tells Jeremiah to our emotional eating. When we turn to food to control our emotions, we leave God's well of living water and go to a leaky vessel believing it will satisfy. What we encounter is a broken source that cannot hold or provide satisfaction.

As I think about these truths, I am humbled even more by how much God loves us and desires a relationship with us. All through the Bible, we see the push and pull of the surrender God wants from us and the ultimate fulfillment that comes from that surrender. We push God away in the attempt to gain our own fulfillment and turn to our broken cisterns, yet God pulls us back into relationship by His tenacious grace.

He tells us that if we trust in people, especially our own hearts, we will dwell in the parched places of our wilderness — an uninhabited salt land where we will forever seek and thirst without relief. If we place our trust in Him, we will be blessed:

> Blessed is the man who trusts in the Lord,
> whose trust is the Lord.
> He is like a tree planted by water,
> that sends out its roots by the stream,
> and does not fear when heat comes,
> for its leaves remain green,
> and is not anxious in the year of drought,
> for it does not cease to bear fruit.
> —Jeremiah 17:7–8 (ESV)

I can't help but see God's tenacious grace all over these verses. He gives us a continual source of living water that produces and sustains life.

When it comes time to fuel our bodies physically, how can we choose healthy food if we aren't fueled up spiritually? If we are trying to control or reinforce our emotions, how can we take those emotions to Christ? We honor God with our bodies by staying fueled with Christ.

Take a few minutes and study what God promises in these verses:

- Matthew 5:6 tells us we are blessed when we hunger and thirst for Christ, and He will satisfy.

- John 6:33–35 tells us He is so satisfying that when we turn to Him, we won't even feel a spiritual hunger and thirst. This promise holds water — no broken cistern here.

GOING DEEPER

1. As we have established, emotional eating is idolatry. How is God humbling and teaching you in your wilderness of discipline?

2. What are the most common thoughts that lead to emotions that trigger you to emotionally eat?

3. What circumstances are you focusing on that cause you to feel spiritual hunger (hopelessness and a lack of satisfaction)?

OWNING TRUTH

*   Feelings are like toddlers. We can't let them drive our cars, but we can't stuff them in the trunk and ignore them either. What we are thinking on will create emotions within us. To stop these feelings from triggering emotional eating, we must change our thought patterns.

*   Allowing for more time between meals will help us recognize the biological sensations that tell us we are physically hungry.

*   To feed spiritual hunger, we must resolve to turn to God — the only One who can hold satisfaction and fulfillment for us — rather than food, which is unable to do anything other than fuel our physical bodies.

CHAPTER 4

Captive To Your Thoughts or Taking Your Thoughts Captive?

In the famous words of Yoda, "Do. Or do not. There is no try." The same can be said about how we go about overcoming emotional eating. When we say no to something, we simultaneously say yes to something else.

The truth is that we are constantly making deliberate decisions—even if that decision is to avoid making the right decision. Whenever we choose not to work toward our freedom, we choose to stay imprisoned in the idolatry of emotional eating. When we say no to reaching out or accepting help, we choose to go it alone. We decide in the moment, and that's the reality we must own to overcome this struggle.

Intentionality is defined as "the fact of being deliberate or purposive."[9] Christ calls us to live intentionally, and we are deliberately saying no to Christ when we live on autopilot.

1 Timothy 4:15–16 says to "be diligent in these matters; give yourself wholly to them, so that everyone may see your progress. Watch your life and doctrine closely. Persevere in them, because if you do, you will save both yourself and your hearers."

A vital element in overcoming a stronghold is cleaning up your thought life. Your thoughts become your internal dialogue, and they often go too far. You would never say to others the things you say to yourself. When you engage in negative self-dialogue—or as I like to call it, internal hate speech—your inner warrior hears you and is diminished and devalued. You can either call out or cast down courage within your heart. Friend, be one of your first and best advocates, and with boldness and courage start intentionally fighting the lies you're believing. Your mind can either be Satan's playground or God's training ground. God's truth reminds you to take your thoughts captive and make them obedient to Christ (2 Corinthians 10:5).

THE THREE "A"S OF INTENTIONALITY

As God brought me out of my years of willful rebellion and idolatry into freedom, He showed me a three-step approach that helps me overcome emotional eating. Implementing the three "A"s of intentionality allows us to jam the endless cycle of the trigger, eating, and shame phases of the emotional eating cycle (more on this in Part Two). This approach helps us take our thoughts captive, turn to God first, and treat food as fuel for our bodies rather than fulfillment for our hearts.

I would not be walking in the freedom I have today without becoming familiar with the lies Satan brought to the doorstep of my heart. I'm excited to experience more freedom ahead as I continue to hone the skill set of intentional thinking. Read and learn the verses that make up this process: 2 Corinthians 10:5, 2 Peter 1:3, and Philippians 4:8.

1. Analyze Your Thoughts

> We tear down arguments, and every presumption set up
> against the knowledge of God.
>
> —2 Corinthians 10:5a (BSB)

The first thing we must do is analyze our thoughts and the lies we're believing. To analyze means to "examine (something) methodically and in detail, typically in order to explain and interpret it."[10]

We must first ask God to reveal what is going on in our thoughts. Here are three questions to ask if it's hard to clearly identify the lies you're believing: "What am I feeling? What happened that triggered that feeling? What do I think about what happened?" When we answer these questions, we will learn to identify the lies from Satan as we ask God to clearly reveal them.

When Satan lies to us, he wraps up a little truth with a bunch of lies. Remember Satan's strategy of distorting truth and feeding Eve lies, causing her to doubt God's goodness? This was his focus more than the fruit itself, but Eve's lack of intentional thought control easily led her into giving the fruit way more power than God ever intended for it to have. Believing Satan's lies caused Eve to forget God's truth. When we are intentional in analyzing our thoughts, God helps us to identify the lies and implement His truth. It's important to know God's truth so we can more easily draw from it during Satan's attacks.

Ask God to reveal the specific lies that Satan is feeding you. Once you have identified the lies, it's time to implement the second step.

2. Annihilate Satan's Lies

> We take captive every thought to make it obedient to Christ.
> —2 Corinthians 10:5b (BSB)

Next, we will annihilate the lies we identified by taking our thoughts captive. To take something captive is to take away its freedom. Satan is the father of lies, and he gives his lies the freedom to enslave us. When we take his lies captive, we take that freedom away.

We must claim ownership of the freedom we have in Christ to fight against Satan's lies and not give into temptation. Galatians 5:1 tells us that Jesus died for our freedom, so we are to own that freedom and not allow Satan's lies to take us captive again and lead us back under the heavy yoke of slavery to the sin of idolatry.

We then make the lies from Satan bow down to Christ. The most powerful thing we can do to obliterate the power of Satan's lies over us is to command them to get in line with God's truth.

Satan and his lies will always be at your doorstep until you are at home, in Heaven, with Jesus. That doesn't mean, however, that you have no other option than to let those lies have free range in your mind and heart. Willfully and with intention, tell Satan that you reject each specific lie in Jesus' name and then pray and give God the lie. Ask Him to heal the damage and restore a strong spirit within you. Ask God to reveal specific truths from His Word to replace the lies from Satan. Once you have claimed victory in captivating your thoughts and identified key truths from God's Word, you move onto step three.

3. Appropriate Jesus' Truth.

> His divine power has given us everything we need for life and godliness through the knowledge of Him who called us by His own glory and excellence.
> —2 Peter 1:3 (BSB)

Now it's time to appropriate the truth of Jesus. The power that comes with knowing the truth of Jesus Christ sets us free when we cling to and use it. To appropriate something means to take it for one's own use. God tells us we have everything we need. We lack nothing. Psalm 34:9 (ESV) tells us, "Oh, fear

the Lord, you his saints, for those who fear him have no lack!"
Satan lied to Eve in the garden, implying that she lacked wisdom. Through knowing Jesus as our personal Savior, we have
the power to be diligent, virtuous, knowledgeable, temperate,
patient, godly, kind, and generous. These are some specific
promises that are direct results of us being partakers in this
divine power through salvation.

Every time we study God's Word and hide it in our hearts,
we know more truth so we can appropriate more of His truth.
He tells us what to think on in Philippians 4:8. We must replace
the lies with the truth! When we overcome a lie that has been
a large factor in our struggles, there is an empty space left that
must be filled. If we aren't intentional in filling it with godly
thoughts like those in Philippians, we will turn back to old
familiar thoughts that made up the walls of our strongholds.
Once you take God's truth and the power of His Holy Spirit
and use it in your decision-making, your life will be a reflection
of God's power.

OUT WITH THE OLD, IN WITH THE NEW

Let's practice the first A and analyze some common lies we
believe regarding emotional eating. Here are 10 lies I identified
as I analyzed my thoughts. This is a good place to start, but I
encourage you to take the time and write out more specific lies
you believe that keep you trapped. We can't overcome lies we
haven't identified.

- Analyzing Your Thoughts Lie #1: Food can fill a void
  within my heart and provide protection and companionship, numb the pain, bring happiness, and meet any
  other emotional need I have.

- Analyzing Your Thoughts Lie #2: I'm not emotionally
  eating. There's no real emotion attached to this; I just
  want to eat. I'm free to make my own choices.

- Analyzing Your Thoughts Lie #3: I'm in control. I'm choosing to eat this, and I can start making better decisions tomorrow.

- Analyzing Your Thoughts Lie #4: Emotional eating isn't a sin. At least I'm not like someone else who committed the sin of _____.

- Analyzing Your Thoughts Lie #5: It really doesn't matter. It's only this one time. It won't hurt anything or make a real impact.

- Analyzing Your Thoughts Lie #6: Everyone else can eat what they want. I'm the only one struggling with this.

- Analyzing Your Thoughts Lie #7: I'm not worth much if I don't look a certain way or weigh a certain amount. Skinny equals beautiful.

- Analyzing Your Thoughts Lie #8: I must be thin before I can be happy or receive any blessings in life.

- Analyzing Your Thoughts Lie #9: I'm so fat, ugly, lazy, and gross. I have the wrong shape, wrong eye color, wrong hair, etc.

- Analyzing Your Thoughts Lie #10: I can't overcome this because I keep messing up. Why try?

Now that we have identified some lies through the analyze step, let's apply the second step and annihilate these lies with God's truth. It's important to let God's Word be what it is: the sword of the Spirit. It has more power to cut through Satan's lies than anything we could ever think of. Here are some truths from God's Word that take captive the lies above:

- Annihilating Satan's Lie #1: "And my God will meet all your needs according to the riches of his glory in Christ Jesus" (Philippians 4:19).

- Annihilating Satan's Lie #2: "You, however, are controlled not by the flesh, but by the Spirit, if the Spirit of God lives in you. And if anyone does not have the Spirit of Christ, he does not belong to Christ" (Romans 8:9, BSB).

- Annihilating Satan's Lie #3: "They tested God in their heart by demanding the food they craved" (Psalm 78:18, ESV).

- Annihilating Satan's Lie #4: "The heart is deceitful above all things, and desperately sick; who can understand it?" (Jeremiah 17:9, ESV).

- Annihilating Satan's Lie #5: "I appeal to you therefore, brothers, by the mercies of God, to present your bodies as a living sacrifice, holy and acceptable to God, which is your spiritual worship" (Romans 12:1, ESV).

- Annihilating Satan's Lie #6: "No temptation has overtaken you that is not common to man. God is faithful, and he will not let you be tempted beyond your ability, but with the temptation he will also provide the way of escape, that you may be able to endure it" (1 Corinthians 10:13, ESV).

- Annihilating Satan's Lie #7: "For the Lord sees not as man sees: man looks on the outward appearance, but the Lord looks on the heart" (1 Sam 16:7b, ESV).

- Annihilating Satan's Lie #8: "Food will not commend us to God. We are no worse off if we do not eat, and no better off if we do" (1 Corinthians 8:8, ESV).

- Annihilating Satan's Lie #9: "For you formed my inward parts; you knitted me together in my mother's womb. I praise you, for I am fearfully and wonderfully made. Wonderful are your works; my soul knows it very well. My frame was not hidden from you, when I was being made in secret, intricately woven in the depths of the earth. Your eyes saw my unformed substance; in your book were written, every one of them, the days that were formed for me, when as yet there was none of them" (Psalm 139:13–16, ESV).

- Annihilating Satan's Lie #10: "He found him in a desert land, and in the howling waste of the wilderness; he encircled him, he cared for him, he kept him as the apple of his eye. Like an eagle that stirs up its nest, that flutters over its young, spreading out its wings, catching them, bearing them on its pinions, the Lord alone guided him, no foreign god was with him" (Deuteronomy 32:10–12, ESV).

Applying the third step, let's take the truths that annihilated the lies of Satan above and appropriate them — take them and use them for our own benefit.

- Appropriating Jesus' Truth for Lie #1: Through Jesus, I lack nothing. I need to ask Him to satisfy my needs and remind myself that food cannot touch my heart emotionally.

- Appropriating Jesus' Truth for Lie #2: Because I am in a relationship with Christ, I am not controlled by the flesh unless I willingly give the desires of my flesh the power to control me. If I believe I am free to make my own choices and just eat what I want without stewarding my body, I am being controlled by the flesh and I am not surrendered to the Spirit of God living within me.

- Appropriating Jesus' Truth for Lie #3: When I test God's discipline by demanding to go and seek my own fulfillment through food, I am prideful and choosing idolatry.

- Appropriating Jesus' Truth for Lie #4: I think I am in control, but if I can't start making the better decisions immediately, I am not in control. I can't let my heart deceive me.

- Appropriating Jesus' Truth for Lie #5: When I live as a sacrifice to Holy God, I sacrifice my "right" to make my own choices out of selfish desire. It does matter, and it will make a real impact.

- Appropriating Jesus' Truth for Lie #6: I am not the only one who struggles with this. Not everyone can eat what they want. I assume they can and react to that assumption by isolating my own pain. When I surrender to the fact that I will always need to keep my emotional appetite in check, I will move with the current of freedom instead of against it.

- Appropriating Jesus' Truth for Lie #7: God says I am worth Jesus giving up His life on the cross to purchase my freedom. My worth does not come from how I look, but from who I am as His creation. When I limit my standard of worth and value to looks, actions, and other's opinions, I disagree with God's truth and limit my experience of His freedom.

- Appropriating Jesus' Truth for Lie #8: God doesn't wait till I have it all together to bless me. His pursuit of me in the middle of my mess is my biggest blessing. As I reach new points of growth in my heart and mind, God will bring new blessings to strengthen me. Blessings, just as much as trials, are meant to make me more Christlike every day. God doesn't give a blessing without a purpose attached to it. He doesn't check off my "ready for a blessing now" list either.

- Appropriating Jesus' Truth for Lie #9: God knew exactly what He was doing when He created me. There is no part of me that is a mistake. When I look in a mirror and see added weight as an outward result of inward idolatry, there is wisdom is owning responsibility for what I have added to God's creation. I can't take the consequences of my lack of stewardship and put it in the category of God's mistake. He made me with respect and wonder!

- Appropriating Jesus' Truth for Lie #10: When this journey gets overwhelming at times and I feel like I am losing strength, I will remember it is God who finds me where I am and cares for me. He still loves and approves of me and spreads His wings of protection, guidance, and discipline over me. If I would surrender to His power and ability and stop worshipping my selfish desires and food, I could really experience God for who He is. I would then continue to gain more ground in my journey to freedom.

As we learn these truths, we show ourselves to be disciples of Christ—growing, changing, and being molded in His likeness. Then and only then can these truths set us free as it tells us in John 8:31–32. We must cling to His truths as if we were clinging to the edge of a cliff.

The King of Kings calls us beautiful and says He is enthralled with our beauty (Psalm 45:11). Let's not limit beauty to what society says it is. Let's learn to settle into that beauty of becoming more like Christ and loving who God made us to be. Let's honor Him by reminding ourselves that through Jesus' blood on the cross, God made us rich in righteousness. This means we can choose rightly and live a life of godliness by presenting our bodies as living sacrifices, which is our spiritual act of worship.

It's time to accept responsibility by being intentional in taking thoughts captive and analyzing them, annihilating Satan's lies, and appropriating Jesus' truth.

GOING DEEPER

Let's put the three As of intentionality into practice. Write out one specific thought that is frequently a part of your internal dialogue regarding your struggle with food and put it through this process:

1. Analyze the thought (tear down arguments and every presumption set up against the knowledge of God). Pray and ask God to reveal truth and lies. What normally happens before this thought enters your mind? How does it make you feel?

    A. What is the truth?

    B. What is the lie?

2. Annihilate the lie (take captive every thought to make it obedient to Christ). Now that you have identified the lie, take that lie and tell Satan you reject it in Jesus' name. Visualize yourself taking power back from Satan and remind him your mind will not be his playground. Take that lie and write out a prayer about your choice to place it in God's hands. Ask Him to heal what has been broken or damaged by that lie. Choose to trust in God's truth.

    A. Reject the lie.

    B. Place it in God's hands.

3. Appropriate the truth of Jesus Christ (His divine power has given you everything you need for life and godliness through the knowledge of Him who called you by His own glory and excellence). We have everything we need at our fingertips through the Holy Spirit. He tells us what to think on in Philippians 4:8. We must replace the lies with the truth! If you have a personal relationship with Jesus Christ, you have the presence of the Holy Spirit within you, and with that comes all the power and fruits of His Spirit. Choose to act accordingly.

A. Make the choice to apply truth.

B. Remind yourself the lie has no more power.

OWNING TRUTH

- For us to overcome a stronghold, it's important that we clean up our thought lives.

- 2 Corinthians 10:5, 2 Peter 1:3, and Philippians 4:8 are our blueprints for having intentional thought control.

- If we are struggling to believe God's truth, we can still choose to act the way we would if we really did trust Him. This obedience allows us to have opportunities to experience His faithfulness is ways we wouldn't have seen in rebellion.

PART TWO:

The Emotional Eating Cycle

CHAPTER 5

The Trigger Phase

Whenever I reach a certain level of exhaustion — either physically or mentally — I cry. Not like a tear running down my cheek, but the actual ugly cry. I've been this way my whole life. As a young girl, I'd lay in bed many nights with my poor mother listening to me cry about how life was crumbling down around me. She would tell me I was just tired and to go to sleep. Well, that would make me mad. I just knew that my world truly was falling apart in those moments. But I always woke up the next morning and, miraculously, my world was back together again.

Fast forward to one night in my early twenties. I had finished speaking at a retreat, and my mom, my dear friend, and I were in the basement of my parents' house rehashing the whole thing. I was beyond exhausted and fell asleep. About 15 minutes later, I woke up and apologized for drifting off to sleep. I immediately burst into tears as I mumbled, "I'm so tired," and we all laughed. It was clear that even as an adult, my emotional reaction of tears was my body's way of alerting me that it needed rest — not just take an afternoon off and slow down but actually sleep. Hopefully, this is an endearing quality to my friends and family who know that when I'm beyond exhausted, the waterworks will start running.

Just as being exhausted can magnify the tough things in life and make them feel unbearable, Satan's attacks regarding my emotional eating are stronger when I'm tired. He knows that's when I'm at my weakest. That's why it's vital that we discover our vulnerable places and the triggers that trip us up.

The starting point of our habitual eating patterns is the trigger phase. We tend to breeze past this phase when we are mentally on autopilot. To better understand what it means to be "triggered" to emotionally eat, let's unpack the concept.

The word *trigger* is a noun that is defined as "a small device that releases a spring or catch and so sets off a mechanism, especially to fire a gun."[11] There are two other nouns from that definition I want to focus on: *device* and *mechanism*. A device is a plan, scheme, or trick with a particular aim.[12] A mechanism is a natural or established process by which something takes place or is brought about.[13] When applying these definitions to emotional eating, we can say that Satan uses lies and negative thoughts (trigger schemes) attached to nouns (people, places, or things) that release belief systems in our hearts (the spring or catch) to set off an established process of turning to food to cope instead of turning to God (a mechanism).

TRIGGER ZONES

We learned how to live intentionally and discern which type of hunger we are feeling at any given moment: emotional, physical, or spiritual. Those are the same three areas in which we are triggered. External triggers are things like people, certain restaurants, events, items, food itself, or anything that reminds us of old emotional eating attachments. Internal triggers are the thoughts and emotions we leave unchecked. We feel these external and internal triggers in the painful or uncomfortable places of our hearts caused by trauma or hard life circumstances. We eat because of what we believe about our painful experiences, not just because we went through them.

Let's identify some known triggers to help you get the ball rolling. Think about any circumstances, thoughts, and feelings that cause you to eat emotionally, then list them in your journal. Make a chart like mine below. Every time you eat emotionally, write down the food you choose. Then retrace your steps — write down what you felt and the thoughts you had before eating. Now, what triggered those thoughts and feelings?

Triggers can cover a wide range of things, so try not to record general examples like stress, tiredness, or loneliness. Instead, dig deeper and identify what specifically made you feel stressed, tired, or lonely. Once you have established the trigger, write down your feelings and thoughts as you were eating and after you finished. Look up "feeling words" online and you'll find a lot of charts that categorize feelings from low to high intensity. Print out a chart that you like and keep it somewhere you can easily access. These word lists and charts will help you expand your emotional vocabulary. This will help you identify more triggers and become more aware of your feelings.

Triggers	Food I Chose	Feelings and Thoughts Before Eating	Feelings and Thoughts While Eating	Feelings and Thoughts After Eating
Watching TV at night	Pizza	I was lonely; wished I had someone there to cuddle up with. I was tired; wished I had a husband to talk over the day's events with.	Tasted good; it was warm. Something to do other than sitting alone watching TV. I didn't feel alone anymore.	I should have just gone to bed. My stomach is upset now. I can't believe I thought pizza was a substitute for companionship.

PHYSICAL TRIGGER ZONE

Life consists of up and down moments, but when our lifestyle is pushing those up and down swings out of balance, it affects our decision-making when we need to say no to food and yes to God along with other healthy coping mechanisms. Along this journey, we've focused on the spiritual position of our hearts, and while that is the most important factor in why we emotionally eat, it isn't the only factor. We have a responsibility to steward the bodies God gave us. However, most of us run ourselves into the ground with busyness or are overly stressed because of avoiding responsibilities, and we allow fear and negative thought patterns to take root. When we do this, our bodies respond on a biological level.

Homeostasis is a biological term that describes how our autonomic nervous system remains stable and in balance. The autonomic nervous system branches off into the parasympathetic and sympathetic systems. To remain in homeostasis, these two systems coordinate responses to external factors that threaten to disrupt normal function. Let's take a deeper look at each of these.

Fight or Flight Mode

The sympathetic system is the military for our bodies. It has three main functions: regulate body temperature, manage the cardiovascular system, and implement the fight or flight response. Its regulatory and management functions are homeostatic in nature, meaning it works to keep our bodies in homeostasis.

The part of this system that can do a lot of damage (when consistently implemented) is the fight or flight response. This is the function that kicks in when external factors attempt to disrupt homeostasis. When the brain registers danger or a potential threat, it triggers this fight or flight response. When this response is activated, the sympathetic system takes on a catabolic nature, which means the body begins a molecular breakdown process.

Let's say you're hiking out in the woods and a bear comes lumbering around a bend in the path. Your fight or flight response kicks in automatically. Stored energy is mobilized to provide your brain with glucose and your muscles with fatty acids. The thyroid and adrenal glands (which create energy) are activated. Not only do you feel an extra dose of energy, but also your heart rate and blood pressure increase. Your lungs dilate to increase oxygen flow to the blood (this is why some people hyperventilate during panic attacks). Freshly oxygenated blood gets shunted to your muscles, creating a cold sensation. Your pupils dilate to see more of what's happening around you. At this point, your body is ready to either fight the bear or run away from it. The fight or flight response is a gift that God has given us as a survival tool. Without this response, we wouldn't have the instinct to protect ourselves.

But Satan always creeps into the areas that we wouldn't think could be used as spiritual attacks against us. In these physical areas, he can twist what God made for good and use it for bad. He is only able to do this when we are not living intentionally, allowing these attacks to go under the radar.

Satan can use this emergency response against us by luring us into a constant state of stress, panic, or anxiety (triggers). When we live with overbooked schedules, lack of sleep, and unhealthy eating habits, our bodies go into defense mode and deploy the military (fight or flight response) to support this heightened state. We act like the Energizer Bunny, but with a faulty battery. In the same way that our pupils dilate to see our surroundings, we tend to focus on others in comparison, and we can get overwhelmed thinking of everything on our "plates." The longer we stay here, the more intense the response grows.

These high peaks of the sympathetic system's fight or flight response are one reason we see many people suffering from high blood pressure, heart attacks, panic attacks, and strokes. An overly busy life full of fear, anxiety, anger, and stress is like being attacked by a bear 24 hours a day, 7 days a week. We were not designed to remain in this emergency state long term, so our bodies hit a wall — we either get sick, have breakdowns, or fall into depression. When this happens, we have crossed over to the low peaks of the parasympathetic system.

Rest and Digest Mode

If the sympathetic system is our bodies' military, the parasympathetic system is the relief effort. This relief is known as the "rest and digest" mode. It also has three main functions: restore the body back to homeostasis after the fight or flight response has been implemented, stimulate gastrointestinal functions, and conserve energy. After the body has implemented the fight or flight response, our parasympathetic system is intended to restore it, but if there are high levels of stress and anxiety, it doesn't get the chance to do so. Therefore, this mode is not able to fully do its job—leaving our bodies in a constant state of survival.

When restoring the body, the parasympathetic system decreases the heart rate, constricts the pupils to focus the eye for near vision again, and contracts the lungs to lessen the intensity of oxygen flow. This system also stimulates GI functions and empties the bladder and bowels. This is why people tend to have an upset stomach after a stressful encounter.

The parasympathetic system is anabolic in nature, which means the body begins a molecular rebuilding process. It focuses on healing, regenerating, and nourishing the body. It uses nutrients from our food to repair and rebuild muscles and cells as well as support organ function. This is why it's vital that we choose healthy food with the nutrients our bodies need. We can be our bodies' advocates instead of their enemies.

The thing to note about this system is that it is dominant in relaxed individuals. Rest, relaxation, and focusing on God's truth can help activate this mode. Living intentionally and not allowing the stresses of life to create faulty belief systems helps us not to live in the reactive mode of the fight or flight response, which can tear our bodies down. Striving to operate from this rest and digest mode allows our bodies to focus more time and energy on the repairing, resting, and restoring processes. As a part of this mode's restoring functions, we can reduce our focus (like the pupils constricting); instead of comparing ourselves to others, we target our focus on God's purpose in our lives.

But Satan can use this relief effort against us too. Through passive activities like remaining immobile due to depressive thoughts, disassociation, and emotional or physical withdrawal, we get out of balance within the parasympathetic system. Feelings such as hopelessness, despair, and shame can be present in this mode. Other aspects of lethargy and boredom can be present as well. These emotions and many more cause their own anxiety because life keeps moving even if we aren't.

Here, in the low points of this system, we have a strong pull toward emotional eating. A false belief accompanies these low points that tells us we *can't* say no to food. It gives Satan plenty of opportunities to fill our heads with lies and negative dialog. The longer we stay in the negative tailspin of unchecked thoughts, the more depression increases the intensity of our triggers, and we continue to trend downward.

The Pendulum Swing

I once heard a military man say that his mind was his pilot and his body was the machine. If our minds are our pilots, the state of our bodies will reflect our thoughts. As our mindsets determine our emotions, our bodies will manifest the system we are operating on—the fight or flight or the rest and digest. There is no peace when we are pulled back and forth on the leash of our feelings. We swing back and forth between each system until we flatline.

> There is no peace when we are pulled back and forth on the leash of our feelings.

Your flatlines may show in apathy, letting yourself go, eating disorders, anxiety disorders, addictions, sickness, job loss, loss of relationships, spiritual depletion, and more. To avoid flatlining, you must stop periodically and take your emotional temperature.

High-intensity emotions that make you feel "revved up" (stress, anger, anxiety, tension) tell you that you're most likely out of balance with the sympathetic fight or flight mode, and your emotions are in the driver's seat. To balance it, first spiritually refill and rest. To rest emotionally and physically, try making priorities, managing your time, pampering yourself, seeking out help, taking power naps, and engaging in other refreshing activities.

Low-intensity emotions that make you feel drugged or in a fog (depression, boredom, exhaustion, stress from procrastination) tell you that you're most likely out of balance with the parasympathetic rest and digest mode. The solution to balance it? Seek God through prayer and Bible study. Along with that, it's important to get up and walk, work out, complete some housework, go to the coffee shop, read a stimulating book, and get help to start accomplishing things on your to-do list.

The sympathetic will always take precedence over the parasympathetic branch because survival takes priority over relaxation. The fight or flight mode powerfully inhibits the rest and digest system. This is a great emergency system God has instilled within us, but if unmanaged, it creates an intense pendulum swing that can drop us in the emotional eating cycle every time. For example, when we are stressed out and constantly on the go, the sympathetic system's fight or flight response suppresses our appetite (since appetite is a function of the parasympathetic system) so it's harder to recognize true physical hunger. This makes it so much easier to eat emotionally because we either eat as a response to the stress rather than the physical hunger or restrict eating because of the stress and then end up binging once we do feel the hunger signals.

Restrictive types of emotional eaters consistently live in a mindset of fear attached to food and have acclimated to the physical feeling of hunger. The hunger signals have been rewired mentally and associated with success in controlling their fear rather than the intended prompt to seek fuel for a healthy body. Whether you're binging or restricting, the fight or flight response is functioning too long past its intended purpose.

Operating within the fight or flight mode is normal these days due to our fast-paced culture. This has increased our stress levels, yet our society is also more sedentary than ever before — giving us little opportunity to burn off the excess energy from stress. Our bodies are either revved up and stimulated with low levels of rest and self-care or immobile and unstimulated with high levels of anxiety. We find little balance in-between. The goal is to remain in homeostasis, riding the ups and downs of life, practicing healthy coping skills, and knowing we serve a big God who is over it all.

Which mode are you in most often? What circumstances typically occur before you emotionally eat? These circumstances trigger the thought patterns that lead you to emotionally eat. Take a few minutes to think through these questions, and my hope is you will start identifying some patterns and events.

EMOTIONAL TRIGGER ZONE

The two systems we've studied play a huge role in the physical trigger zone. However, we must look at some other contributing factors that lead us to the high points of the fight or flight response and the low points of the rest and digest mode.

Fear

First, we need to talk about fear — a major emotional eating trigger for many. Emotions come from a state of mind, so when we look at fear as one of the prominent emotions that trigger emotional eating, we must start with our thoughts. Singles can have fears about their future and whether or not they will have the family they desire. Married couples who want children can have fears about whether or not they'll conceive. Parents can have fears about the safety of their children. Anyone can have fears about their financial troubles, working people have fears about their jobs, students have fears about their studies, etc.

Chronic thought patterns of fear and anxiety lead our bodies to trigger the fight or flight response. This creates a lack of emotional management within a person as thoughts run rampant in their mind. When this happens, confusion always accompanies anxiety. They feel a lack of direction because the thoughts create space for frustration, unmet expectations, and anger.

In Matthew 6:25–34, God tells us not to worry about anything, but in everything go to Him with prayer. Let's focus on the solution that works—keeping our focus on the things of Christ. Verse 33 has been a beacon of hope for me throughout the years. Jesus reminds us that if we seek out God and the things of His kingdom first, He will take care of all the rest. We still do our part, but we leave the results and the worry in His hands.

As I was coming out of my rebellious years, this verse led me through the fears of not being able to truly change, rebuild my reputation, restore relationships, or stay consistent with the work it takes to heal and grow. Jesus impressed on my heart that if I just got face-to-face with Him daily in His Word and in prayer, He would lead me to new levels of freedom. Being in fellowship with other believers and intentionally surrendering my desires to make room for His were also vital parts of my healing.

Our actions reflect the level of worry in our hearts. They also reflect the amount of trust we have in God. He reassures us in Psalm 46:10 that He will calm the chaos in our hearts, and we can know that He is God.

Trauma

Trauma is a very common emotional trigger and can cause a lot of emotional chaos. Trauma is defined as "a physical injury or a deeply distressing or disturbing experience: emotional shock following a stressful event or a physical injury, which may be associated with physical shock."[14] I know that my childhood trauma brought on shame, fear of being myself, confusion as to my role in people's lives, powerlessness to say no or change the outcome of any situation, and anxiety about being alone. If you have endured any type of trauma, please seek help and godly counsel to work through it and allow God to heal your heart wounds as well as your brain's established trauma responses.

When we go through trauma, we tend to attach our need for emotional security and love to someone or something. Once we do this, a whole lineup of destructive behaviors results so as to keep that security in place. Doing intense introspection to identify the places and people I attached my emotional security to (sometimes from a young age) wasn't easy, and it didn't happen overnight. It took a few years to get to the deep roots of my faulty belief systems and identify that I had attached to my brother, food, and men.

Throughout my teen years, the pain in my heart was like a pot of water on the stovetop slowly heating up to a boil. My coping mechanisms with men and food were simmering under the surface but hadn't quite boiled over yet. I had a few rebellious moments, of course, but I was so protected by the identity of "little sister" that I didn't need food or a romantic relationship as much; my focus was on meeting others' needs rather than getting mine met. It wasn't until I lost the closeness with my brother and could no longer put him in the savior role that food and men boiled over and took the savior roles in my heart.

Whenever I felt insecure about my worth, I would place the power to make me feel worthy in the hands of a man (romantically), or I would try to regain the old closeness with my brother. When those failed me, I would use food as an external way to feel in control since I was unable to control my relationships. These were easily interchangeable. Because of the lack of security I felt with my brother, I leaned into men. When I felt insecure with men, I would lean back into my brother. Either way, I had the opportunity to hide who I really was. If I could feel in control of either relationship, I wouldn't feel alone and forced to face the deeper wounds of my heart — the reality that I felt worthless as the Jenna God created me to be. I didn't even know who that was after so many years of hiding.

So much of our struggle with food comes from our struggle with pain, and when triggers lay our wounds bare, we don't always react as we'd want to. During these painful times, we don't stop long enough to address the pain but instead continue to react from our triggered emotions. These reactions include turning to food, relationships, substances, control, and so much more. I stayed in this reaction zone for so long and needed to learn how to identify and address the emotions and then choose how best to respond.

God has taught me to put "parentheses" around my pain so I can deal with it instead of it dealing with me. In writing, parentheses set off additional information (like this). A set of parentheses includes an opening parenthesis and a closing parenthesis. Putting parentheses around my pain means that I begin by making a clear decision to *open* a time of going to God in prayer where I intentionally give myself space to be vulnerable and allow God to meet me in the middle of my pain. There, He can do the healing work only He is capable of doing. During this time, I deal with the raw emotions, thoughts, and — most importantly — God's truth. Sometimes, the only thing I can do is weep at the feet of Jesus because of my pain and choose to trust He's holding me together.

After a bit, I make a clear decision to *close* that time with God. This is where I intentionally leave the pain at His feet and in His hands. I remind myself that I can go back and deal with it with Jesus at any time because my heart and my pain are in the safest, most healing place with Him. This intentional placement of parameters around the hurt that triggers me to emotionally eat helps me not to be ruled by my emotions and just react once I'm triggered.

We must remember that — for most of us — the trauma we experienced is no longer happening, other than what we choose to relive emotionally. For those who are still in the middle of being traumatized in any way, please reach out for help. I pray for your deliverance from your situation.

What I have learned through my experience is that once we are out of our traumatic situation, we must realize that we are making choices today that are being dictated by something that is no longer happening. We are engaging with our perception of how the trauma has defined us. We must take back our power from the trauma and establish new definitions of our worth. We need to leave behind the victim mentality that we are powerless to help ourselves, get some good counseling, and receive the help Jesus offers through a relationship with Him.

No Longer Victims

Some of you have gone through a life-changing event such as a pregnancy, car accident, broken relationship, sickness, or location change. Either positive or negative events were the beginning of your emotional eating, and something inside of you was either lost, taken from you, given up, or broken. In those moments, you might have developed a victim mentality that you still aren't aware of.

Emotional eating triggers include daily stress, how you grade yourself as a mom, relationship status, kids, marital issues, money issues, and so much more. No matter the origin of the triggers, we all deal with the emotional pull to escape or reinforce our negative emotions with food.

When you're triggered, you may find yourself justifying your decision to give in—you believe that you have the "right" because of what you have gone through. You may even feel powerless against the craving for food. This, my friend, is the victim mentality. We have a mighty warrior in Jesus who is our ever-present help in times of trouble, and He has not given us a spirit of fear and powerlessness, but of power, love, and a sound mind as it tells us in 2 Timothy 1:7. We must go to Him in these moments of perceived weakness.

SPIRITUAL TRIGGER ZONE

Why do we question God's greatness and ability to fulfill our hearts? Doesn't He deserve to be worshipped? Last time I checked, food did not create me, die on a cross for my sins, take up residence within my soul, or love me with an everlasting love. Isaiah 45:11–13 reminds us of how God created us, fights to set us free from strongholds, and shows us that He is powerful enough to deliver on His promises. Remember our Persian King, Cyrus? God chose Cyrus to follow Him in His victorious defeat of a foreign army, setting His people free. If God has called us to live in freedom, He will lead us just as He led Cyrus.

We often operate out of fear, frustration, stress, or exhaustion in an attempt to exert control over the circumstances in our lives—and we fail epically at playing God. This is when Satan sneaks in with his lies and twisted truths. He tells us if we grow spiritually then we'll have to give up control, and that threatens the false sense of security we've worked so hard to build. So we avoid seeking out spiritual nurturing. Because we aren't feeding our spiritual hunger, our control tactics (toxic relationships, busyness, overspending, isolation, etc.) are reinforced by our eating, and the downward spiral continues. Growing spiritually does require us giving up control, but it's a surrender that brings freedom, not captivity.

God tells us to not lean into our own understanding, but in everything acknowledge that He is God and He will show us the way. When we press into our own ability to understand things in this life, we are seeking to understand from the limited scope of human comprehension. When we do this, we are left lacking because what God doesn't fill will remain empty. This is the spiritual void that drives us to seek after food.

We keep trying to deal with the symptoms of emotional eating by changing the food we eat or adding exercise to our already overcrowded schedule. While these are vital aspects of getting healthy, if we aren't addressing the reasons we use food instead of God to cope, we will remain in this emotional eating cycle. We must do our main fighting here in the trigger phase. If we don't, the result is a stronghold of emotional eating and a continual lack of trust that God will fulfill our hearts' needs.

Trust is built through trustworthy actions. An honest look at our lack of trust in God reveals that it is *our* actions that aren't trustworthy, not God's. When we don't honor His command to worship Him alone, we don't turn to Him when the hard times hit. We must give God opportunities to show us He is trustworthy instead of going straight to food. Otherwise, we wrongly believe God didn't provide comfort when we never gave Him the chance to begin with.

THERE'S MORE THAN MEETS THE EYE

We often think of emotional eating as only composed of two elements: our lack of willpower and the food itself. In this journey, we're learning that there are many factors at play. Food itself can be one of those external triggers for emotional eating, and we'll unpack that in the eating phase (see the next chapter). But there are other triggers that lead us either to eat more than we should or to feel guilty afterward.

Let's look at our five different senses—sight, sound, taste, smell, and touch—and how they are activated while eating. These senses can be triggers themselves. We may not be feeling an emotional lack at the time our sensory triggers are activated, but when they are, the habitual and ritualistic aspects of emotional eating can easily be ignited, leading us to choose the food.

Sight

When you see advertisements for your favorite restaurant, what thoughts go through your mind? Sometimes, when we see certain foods, we can easily be triggered to think we are hungry. If someone starts talking about food, we can pull up a mental snapshot and be triggered as well. The food photography industry is huge, and there are many tricks to make food look more enticing. The purpose is to bring in more consumers by the mere sight of a dish or product.

Limiting your exposure to these visual triggers is difficult but possible. Oftentimes, while driving home, I used to see the logos for restaurants on the side of the highway and be triggered to want food. I wasn't hungry at all, but when I saw the logos, all of a sudden I wanted to eat. I didn't become physically hungry, but those advertisements served as the tipping point for any triggers that had been building. I had to drive home a different way for a while to overcome this sight trigger.

Our sight triggers can also be activated by what we look at while we are eating emotionally. Neurons in our brains make a connection between our surroundings and the pleasure of food. Whatever or whoever is in view while we eat can create a sort of ritual that we subconsciously seek out for our next food fix. For example, I made a connection with TV and eating. If I am eating and watching TV, I am most likely emotionally eating. The TV itself has become a trigger, and I know if I don't stay intentional and spiritually on guard (while also limiting screen time), I will be triggered to emotionally eat. We must always be on guard and ready to engage in spiritual warfare, but especially when our known triggers are around.

Sound

Sound plays a big role in triggering the ritual of emotional eating. It's likely that when you eat, you're not doing it in silence. You're either in a restaurant hearing the hustle and bustle of people, in front of a television, listening to the radio, or hearing some other noise that drowns out the reality of your thoughts. Someone talking about food, the crinkle of a bag of chips opening, the buzz of a microwave, or the opening of the refrigerator door can all trigger our desire for food.

Even the sound of chewing can invite us to come back for more. There are professional taste testers who put products through multiple rounds of testing to provide companies with feedback on the perfect amount of crunch or crackle in a food product. It's no coincidence that "you can't eat just one."

Taste

The tongue is an amazing organ. We have nerve endings in our taste buds that pick up chemicals in the food we eat and transmit them to our brains as taste. The five tastes are sweet, salty, bitter, sour, and savory. It's no wonder food can taste so good—our tongue was designed to enjoy the taste of food!

It's not a sin to enjoy eating or choose a particular dish simply because we appreciate its taste, but we take a wrong turn when we try to make our hearts enjoy the taste of food. When we indulge in food from a heart of idolatry (we aren't physically hungry to begin with, or we feel like we couldn't say no if we wanted to), we reinforce taste's power over us.

Smell

Odors can connect our brains to memories, triggering pleasant thoughts that correlate with a certain food. In these instances, we need to remind ourselves that we can enjoy the smell attached to the food without having the food itself.

Certain smells can trigger a belief system. The scent of pumpkin spice takes me to the fall season, which is my favorite. This does not trigger me. On the other hand, vanilla scents take me to the winter season, which makes me think of the holidays. Christmas, New Year's, and Valentine's Day are basically the trifecta of triggers when you're single and desiring a husband and family of your own. Vanilla scents trigger me to want emotional support from food because I'm still single and, at times, I fear I will remain single when those seasons come around again. I have to be guarded and fight against temptation—not only the temptation to eat but to believe the lie that I am incomplete if I'm still single during those holidays.

Touch

Our last sense is touch. The feel of food can trigger emotions within us. When I'm needing comfort and grab the bread, its softness feels like a little pillow for my heart to lay on. As I write that, I just laugh to myself thinking how crazy that seems. Unfortunately, when we struggle with emotional eating, we view food in weird ways.

The place where we eat can also act as a touch trigger. If I'm sitting at my kitchen table, I'm not likely to get lost in emotional eating. But curled up on my comfy couch, I'm more likely to go into autopilot, reach for the remote, and emotionally eat.

Everyone operates differently when it comes to triggers and how their brains respond to emotional stimuli, so it's important to understand your senses and which ones create more triggers for you. As you read through each of the senses just now, you might have thought of your favorite foods and found yourself triggered. Guard your mind and know that, although there are thoughts present, that doesn't mean you must follow through in action and give into those triggers.

JAMMING THE FIRING PIN

Now that you've brought your triggers to light, the next step is to put an end to their power over you. We can't control when thoughts come into our minds, but we can control what we do with them. Using our metaphor of a trigger, once a trigger is pulled, the gun will fire—unless the firing pin is jammed or broken. If we are intentional in taking our thoughts captive and asking God to reveal our unique triggers, we can jam Satan's firing pin and stop the unhealthy coping mechanism of emotional eating from igniting within us.

I've found the best way to avoid being triggered is managing my daily routine. I do the investigative work to check and see if there are potential triggers in my schedule, people in my life, thought patterns, etc. before I plunge into my day.

> I've learned that, given the busyness of my life, if I don't spend my mornings with my first love, Jesus, my heart tends to love the chaos of the day as it provides many opportunities for me to be my own god.

First things first—time with God in prayer and His Word is my top priority. I know I need to realign my mind and heart with His truth. This is such a power-ful way to keep Satan's grubby fingers off my triggers for the day. I've learned that, given the busyness of my life, if I don't spend my mornings with my first love, Jesus, my heart tends to love the chaos of the day as it provides many opportunities for me to be my own god.

Some triggers are hard to prevent. We often find ourselves smack dab in the middle of interacting with a person, place, or thing that becomes an unforeseen trigger. Most likely, your feelings will give the alarm that you're being triggered. Immediately, start the process of working through the three As of intentionality.

Here's an example of working through a major trigger: the unhealthy emotional attachment with my brother. I've shared with you that he was my best friend and protector growing up. I had unknowingly given him the savior role to create peace in my heart, but I lost that peace in the years after he got married. During my rebellious years, we didn't really have a relationship and barely ever saw each other.

Once I came out of that downward spiral and started intentionally surrendering my life, pain, and heart to God, I started working at our family business. I worked in a position where my direct boss was none other than my brother. As we worked together, I was surprised by how increasingly insecure I felt around him. Every time we had a conversation, I would fall back into that little sister identity where I told myself it was more important for him to be happy than me. I felt powerless when we had any type of conflict. I wouldn't let myself have a voice, and I was still trying to relate to him as if he were my source of approval and safety.

I would never have thought my brother (my source of security when I was young) could now be a trigger for me. This was *after* a lot of my healing had already happened. I was frustrated with myself and confused by how I felt around him.

I didn't realize my idolatry until God revealed this unhealthy attachment through counseling. I was reminded of it every time I got triggered by him. I analyzed my thoughts surrounding my feelings of insecurity and confusion, linked them to our childhood relationship, and identified and annihilated the lies from Satan that said my brother (or any human) could be my source of approval and safety on a soul level. Then I appropriated the truth that God was the only One capable of providing security for my heart. I pushed through the uncomfortable feelings when I was around my brother and learned to show up fully as myself—healed and secure in Christ. *Me.* I was able to take back the power I had given my brother as my emotional safety net and give that power to Jesus instead. By doing this (along with other heart healing), my dependency on my brother, food, and men have drastically decreased. I'll always need to keep them in check, but I can confidently say I'm walking in freedom from all three of my early idols.

GOING DEEPER

1. What are some of your triggers in each zone: physical, emotional, and spiritual?

2. Whatever your triggers, you are worth the effort it takes to walk in obedience to Jesus. You are valuable, and Jesus wants you living in freedom from this emotional pull of food. It is, after all, why He set you free — for freedom. What do your actions show that you believe you're worth?

3. Romans 5:5-6, 8 shows us what we are worth in God's eyes: "And hope does not put us to shame, because God's love has been poured into our hearts through the Holy Spirit who has been given to us. For while we were still weak, at the right time Christ died for the ungodly. But God shows his love for us in that while we were still sinners, Christ died for us." What does God say you're worth?

OWNING TRUTH:

- God says you are worth His Son's life and the Holy Spirit's home. You are priceless. Your position in Christ demands respect. You are not powerless against the pull of food. You have the power, through the Holy Spirit, to walk out of this prison of emotional eating.

- Both the sympathetic and parasympathetic systems coordinate with each other to keep a balance within our bodies called homeostasis. God is all for balance, and homeostasis can be a physical reflection of a spiritual and emotional balance. Ecclesiastes 7:18 tells us that whoever fears God will avoid all extremes. This fear is a reverence for who God is. Understand that God is bigger than the things making you anxious and causing depression.

- We must use self-control not only to stop emotionally eating but also to be better stewards of our bodies. Self-control is a fruit of the Spirit. Take that fruit and eat *it* when you're tempted to emotionally eat.

CHAPTER 6

The Eating Phase

"**I**'m going to start Monday."

Does this sound familiar? This is the negotiation process that happens after the trigger phase and right before the eating phase. It's where we go back and forth with the thoughts surrounding a pending decision to emotionally eat.

When we're negotiating with Satan, exchanging truth for his lies, we have a choice: either engage in emotional eating as a coping mechanism or turn to God for truth and fulfillment.

Let me explain *coping*. Coping is dealing with something effectively, but when we have unhealthy coping mechanisms, we deal with our emotions ineffectively. Sure, eating handles our emotions temporarily, but it's not a lasting solution.

Identifying what we are trying to cope with is important, but

> Coping is dealing with something effectively, but when we have unhealthy coping mechanisms, we deal with our emotions ineffectively.

after some negotiation with Satan's lies, we go straight to what we believe is our answer: food. We don't do what we *know*. We do what we *believe*. We know God is the answer, but we don't believe He is in these moments, and that is clearly revealed when we turn to food and not Him. We negotiate with Satan for what's quick, easy, and tangible instead of turning to God who satisfies. Surrendering our control and choosing to have faith that God will satisfy are two requirements for overcoming our established unhealthy coping mechanisms.

Can I let you in on a little secret? The longer you negotiate with Satan, the more likely you are to give in to the idolatry of emotional eating. Remember Eve and Satan's conversation in the garden? The key word there is *conversation*. Eve had been walking with God and knew God's voice, His character, and His stance on eating from the tree of the knowledge of good and evil. When Satan approached her about the tree (an issue she had already received instruction about from God), Eve should have stopped and identified Satan's voice as *not* the voice of God, quickly shut him down, and walked away. Instead, she took it upon herself to set Satan straight about the situation, all the while getting more confused by his craftiness.

We must learn to know God's voice so well that when we hear Satan's voice, we don't even let him finish a sentence. The longer Eve negotiated with Satan in the garden, the easier it was for her to sin against God and bring her husband into the sin as well.

THE EMOTIONAL MEAL

To best understand the eating phase, we need to look at how our body responds to food before, during, and after eating. Satan wants to wrap shame around us like a cloak (we'll unpack shame more in the next chapter) by telling us the lie that the only contributing factor in our stronghold of emotional eating is our inability to say no to food. Sadly, society places this stigma on our struggle as well. Understanding emotional eating as an umbrella with many pieces underneath it — like the triggers we unpacked in the last chapter along with the food itself and the shame that follows — will help us deconstruct the stigma, negative connotations, shame, and defeating thoughts. Then we can more easily take on the pieces one bite at a time, so to speak.

Emotionally eating (including restricting and binging) is where we find a temporary answer to our fear, exhaustion, loneliness, etc. When we're on autopilot and following Satan's lead into idolatry, we focus so much on food that the reasons we turned to or avoided the food fade into the background. This is when we need to put a magnifying glass over what we are trying to cope with. We do this by analyzing what is happening around us, our thoughts and feelings, and how our bodies respond. Take a few moments and write out what happens in your eating phase. Then keep track the next handful of times you engage in emotional eating. For restrictive types, it will help you to identify what you turn to instead of food while you're actively in a restrictive mindset.

The eating phase is the hardest area when it comes to identifying what thoughts and emotions are going on within us and what triggered us to eat. But this phase is the most important to understand. We are not fueling our bodies during this eating phase; we are attempting to feed or control our emotions. This is where we have to come to grips with the reality that we believe food can be our emotional "fix-it" tool.

For example, busyness is one area where we attempt to feed our emotions. We have to be intentional in planning our activities and not letting them plan us. The exhaustion from busyness can easily present opportunities to justify convenient but unhealthy meals. Food that is full of empty calories doesn't give us lasting energy but rather forces our bodies to use extra energy to break it down. The problem is we aren't replenishing that energy because we're too busy, and we eat another empty-calorie meal later. We walk around feeling tired all the time because of this pattern. We have high blood sugar spikes followed by crashes that leave us craving more of the processed food that gave us the quick spike. This creates a physical addiction to processed food. When events or people trigger us to eat emotionally, the food we choose reinforces our feelings and thoughts attached to those circumstances. This creates an emotional addiction with food at the center.

For those who struggle with restrictive eating, staying busy can be a way to avoid food. In this case, fear of what food can do to your body is running the show and leaving you with less energy. This can create an addiction to other things that give you a sense of control, giving you the temporary feeling of fixing the emotions connected to food.

When you get this "fix," do you sometimes feel like you aren't fully present or self-aware? After being triggered and avoiding food or turning to it emotionally, many of us feel as though we've been mentally hijacked; the experience is a blur. The reason we aren't fully engaged mentally is that we are fully engaged emotionally. This feeding of our emotional state has crossed into an addictive or dependent need for food or for the things chosen while avoiding the food.

This out-of-body experience is accompanied by a sense of euphoria and anesthesia. This is when our amygdala (the pleasure center in our brains) is ignited and our prefrontal cortex (the reasoning center) is inhibited. The more we seek out a food fix for our emotions, the more our pleasure center will be engaged and our ability to reason our way out will be inhibited. Let's look at how the type of food we turn to plays a huge role in reinforcing our dependency on food.

PROCESSED FOODS

Let me guess — you aren't turning to broccoli when you're emotionally eating, are you? From personal experience, I know that you probably turn to processed food filled with additives and chemicals that create a flavor explosion in your mouth. It's vital for you to understand that unhealthy food is only creating more deficits in your emotional state and reinforcing the addictiveness of food.

Food that is processed (not in its original form) has also been designed. These foods start a sensory party in our minds and bodies in order to keep us coming back for more. Keep in mind that junk food and processed food come from companies trying to make a profit. The majority of them are not worried about how their products affect your health—they're thinking about their bottom line.

Junk food is the term we commonly use to refer to cheap food with high levels of calories, sugar, and fat. This type of food has little nutritional value due to having small amounts of vitamins, minerals, fiber, etc.

Do you know how healthy food affects your body? Your gut is comprised of the small and large intestines, and it acts as a second brain because it has numerous nerve endings that connect to the brain. There are so many neurons in the gut that when you eat nutrient-rich foods, they naturally trigger the release of normal levels of hormones and neurotransmitters like GABA, glutamate, dopamine, norepinephrine, and serotonin (the hormones that influence your emotions). This is largely because natural sugar is broken down into glucose within your digestive tract, and one of the places it travels to is your brain. Glucose travels to the part of your brain responsible for rewards, which sends your body a "thank you, come again" message so that you continue to seek out healthy doses of normal sugar found in complex carbohydrates.

Processed junk food also triggers the release of hormones and neurotransmitters like those above, but in abnormally large doses, thus creating an addiction to the chemicals in those processed foods. This keeps you in the destructive cycle of emotional eating.

For example, artificial sweeteners don't travel to the brain's natural reward center; they stimulate the brain's pleasure and desire center. This releases dopamine (pleasure hormone) and triggers serotonin (calming hormone), giving you a euphoric feeling. The chemical sweeteners in processed food ignite the pleasure center the same way alcohol and drugs do in the brain of someone who is addicted to them. To make matters worse, this process inhibits the adrenals from releasing satiety hormones to tell your body you're full, so you're likely to consume more calories than you need and continue indulging.

The result is a cycle of sugar highs and crashes. When we eat processed and artificial sugars, our blood sugar and feel-good hormone levels spike and then suddenly drop, leaving us feeling wiped out and shaky—which makes us search for more sweets to regain that sugar high. And now, we've reached sugar-addiction land.

Because our bodies are hungry, they look for fuel. But if we feed them processed sugar, they increase their potential to consume more calories later in a desperate search for nutritious fuel. This is why there are extremely overweight people who are starving themselves to death.

Let's look at the five main artificial sweeteners that are added to our processed foods:

- Aspartame (Equal): 160-220x sweeter than sugar

- Acesulfame-K: 200x sweeter than sugar

- Saccharin (Sweet'N Low): 200–700x sweeter than sugar

- Sucralose (Splenda): 600x sweeter than sugar

- Neotame: 8,000x sweeter than sugar[15]

These sweeteners are all approved for use in the US, but they are chemically manufactured molecules—they do not exist in nature. We can see how they are much sweeter than sugar, reinforcing a biological addiction to foods that contain them. This increased addiction to junk food causes many health problems that add another layer to our struggle.

We can either allow food to make us sick or allow it to bring healing. Hippocrates said, "Let food be thy medicine and medicine be thy food." In 431 BC, the ancient Greeks didn't have the pharmaceuticals we do now, so they learned about certain foods that assisted healing. Thank God for modern medicine and how it can save lives, but if we are dependent on medicine and do not nourish our bodies with good food, we need to step back and realize we are creating problems at the same time we're trying to fix them. It's the treadmill effect — we're busy going nowhere.

A big part of understanding the eating phase is learning the biology of what's happening. Not only are we emotionally seeking a fix, but also our physical sensations are craving a fix. Our bodies yearn for nutrients but also for the chemical highs they have experienced through the neurotransmission process.

STILL AN OUT

Balance is an essential mindset for me. I have to balance my busyness with downtimes when I can recharge so I stay intentional in all areas, and that requires self-control. Galatians 5:22–23 says, "But the fruit of the Spirit is love, joy, peace, patience, kindness, goodness, faithfulness, gentleness and self-control." God calls us to allow the Holy Spirit to produce the fruit of self-control in us. If we are not letting God into the area of our idolatry issue with food, how can the Holy Spirit produce that fruit within us? The strength to say no needs to come from God's power through us, not our own power. We won't find freedom and balance until we stop going to food (or other "answers") and instead ask God to produce life-changing fruits in our lives.

We learned in the last chapter that emotional eating is a mechanism that is set off by the triggering schemes or thoughts from Satan that become attached to certain people, places, or things specific to our experiences. It's hard to reason our way out of the eating phase.

But thanks to the tenacious grace of God, we can still fight when we are in this eating phase.

1. First, we pray for help and realize we are personifying food as our answer to an emotional issue.

2. Then we clearly identify what it is that we expect the food to do. If we don't know that yet, we ask ourselves what we need emotionally. Companionship, stress-relief,

something to do, and celebration are just a few ideas to start with. We need to take a moment to identify these needs while we are eating.

3. It's important to clearly identify what food will *not* do. For example, food is not a sustainable source of companionship, stress-relief, validation, or affirmation.

4. Focusing on exactly what is happening emotionally and in our thoughts during this phase is vital. Having a sound mind with clarity about our strongholds is one of our mightiest weapons to fight the confusion and deceit of Satan's lies.

5. We must make it clear to ourselves that it no longer makes sense to keep eating the food and *put it down*. We need to make a decision — our choice buttons are not broken! We can drive out of the drive-through line or throw away the remaining piece of pizza. Just because we're in the middle of eating doesn't mean we *have* to keep eating.

Along with doing the mental work it takes to keep our focus on what's going on internally while emotionally eating, we also need to do the spiritual work. I can imagine God asking us, "How long will you turn to food for your hearts' fulfillment and satisfaction when it provides nothing more than a temporary distraction?" Haven't we learned by now that its effects are not lasting, that we have to keep going back for more? It's exhausting, to say the least.

In Jeremiah 31:23–25, God says, "When I bring them back from captivity . . . I will refresh the weary and satisfy the faint." God yearns to bring us out of captivity so He can be the One who refreshes and fulfills us. Friend, isn't it time we let Him? It's not that God needs our permission or that He can't snap us out of it; He's powerful enough to do those things. Just as God gave Eve and Adam the freedom to choose obedience, we also have that choice. We end up resisting God's grace in the moments when He is waiting to give us the full strength to say no to food and yes to Him! He brings us out a few steps and then we run back toward our idol of self and serve Satan's lies on the platter of food for an emotional fix. God patiently and lovingly pursues our hearts to show us the truth.

I know this is a struggle that feels so overwhelming with its ups and downs. The eating phase is the hardest to overcome because this is the heart of our stronghold. It's where we falsely believe we are protected and provided for. Sadly, it's only momentary. Until we stop seeing food for what we want it to be, we won't learn what food *truly* is and what it is not.

Back in the early days of our Tenacious Grace Support Groups, many times I found myself stopping by a fast food restaurant to emotionally eat on the way home. I would feel so defeated because I had just spent time teaching women about these truths and processing thoughts and feelings with them, but I hadn't discovered what food *truly* was and was not for me. However, I was working toward learning that, and I discovered more and more the longer I did the deep emotional work with God.

I had to remind myself that the process of tearing down something I'd spent years reinforcing wasn't going to happen overnight. Working with the women was bringing out my own struggles, and I had to learn how to simultaneously teach truth, own it, and walk in it myself. It was good accountability for me because it kept me from going back into a rebellious mindset of doing what I wanted without care of consequence. The fact I had the group kept me moving forward *through* the struggle instead of stopping *in* another time of struggle.

God is faithful, and He is pursuing your heart. Please let Him reveal what is in your heart during these times of emotional eating. Psalm 139:23 (ESV) says, "Search me, O God, and know my heart! Try me and know my thoughts! And see if there be any grievous way in me, and lead me in the way everlasting!" Don't let Satan's lies make you believe you can't be open and seek God in these moments. He will always meet you in the midst of your sin and lead your heart toward freedom.

God tells us we can find refuge in the shadow of His wings (Psalm 91:4). My desire is that—like a child keeping in step with the shadow of their parent for protection, guidance, and shelter—we will live life in the shadow of His protective faithfulness. Even during moments of emotional eating, you can run to God and ask Him to reveal what you are seeking to gain from food. Remind yourself that even though you are already emotionally eating, it doesn't mean you have failed and therefore should keep on eating. The fact you identified you were emotionally eating shows progress in and of itself. Take that truth and—with boldness—put the food down, walk away, and seek fulfillment in God! He is consistently inviting us to find shelter and refuge in Him. Finding shelter in food pales in comparison to finding shelter in our Creator, Savior, and Counselor. Let's give God the opportunity to shield us from Satan's attacks.

GOING DEEPER

1. Get out your "magnifying glass" and examine your emotional eating experience: what happens, how you feel, what you are thinking, what's happening around you, what foods make you feel which way, and what you want to get out of food. Take a few moments and write out what happens in your eating phase.

2. Our tongue was designed to enjoy the taste of food. We take a wrong turn when we try to make our hearts enjoy the taste of food. What taste do you tend to go for when looking for that emotional fix? How do you think that physical taste plays a part in the emotional aspect of what you're looking for?

3. Create a list that connects specific foods with experiences where you felt secure emotionally.

OWNING TRUTH

• Thanks to the tenacious grace of God, you can still fight when you are in this eating phase:

1. Pray for help and realize you are personifying food as your answer to an emotional issue.

2. Clearly identify what it is that you expect the food to do. If you don't know that yet, ask yourself what you need emotionally. Take a moment to identify these needs while you are eating.

3. Clearly identify what food will *not* do. For example, food is not a sustainable source of companionship, stress-relief, validation, or affirmation.

4. Focus on exactly what is happening emotionally and in your thoughts during this phase.

5. Make it clear to yourself that it no longer makes sense to keep eating the food and *put it down*. Make a decision—your choice button is not broken! Just because you're in the middle of eating doesn't mean you *have* to keep eating.

- Having a sound mind with clarity about our strongholds is one of our biggest weapons to fight the confusion and deceit of Satan's lies. God tells us to ask Him to search our hearts. Take some time and, through prayer, write down what God reveals about your heart.

- God tells us we can find refuge in the shadow of His wings. Finding shelter in food pales in comparison to finding shelter in our Creator, Savior, and Counselor. Let's give God the opportunity to shield us with His faithfulness against Satan's attacks.

CHAPTER 7

The Shame Phase

Shame is the Achilles' heel of our best intentions to overcome this stronghold of idolatry in emotional eating. After a period of restriction or binging, the emotional fix starts to wear off and we arrive at this shame phase. When we don't fight against the shame, we stay in our strongholds and believe we aren't good enough to go to God for help. What we're left with is physical discomfort from an upset stomach and we feel worse emotionally than we did before we ate.

There they are again — the feelings we tried to quiet, the questions we tried to answer — only now with a nice helping of shame on top. We haven't been filled with what our hearts really want, but we did feel full for a small amount of time and distracted with food, which is what we thought was our answer. Yet the ache or distress remains. We feel even more shameful because we are further into the stronghold or we're back in a place we'd walked away from for so long. This leaves an empty space and pushes us to chase again after those moments of feeling full and distracted, secretly hoping it will finally become the answer we're looking for.

Where there is an empty space, Satan will be there ready to fill it with lies of shame and condemnation. We must fill that space with God's truth so there is no room for Satan's deceit. Hebrews 4:16 (BSB) tells us to "approach the throne of grace with confidence, so that we may receive mercy and find grace to help us in our time of need." The purpose of going to the throne of grace is to receive help when we need it—even after we've messed up. The verse doesn't say, "Go to the throne when you have it all together."

While we were at our worst, Christ died for us. We see this in Romans 5:8 where it says, "But God demonstrates his own love for us in this: While we were still sinners, Christ died for us." It comes down to whether we are going to believe all of God's Word or just some of it. When we believe Christ for our salvation, we must believe Christ for His invitation to go to Him when we are in any kind of need. Our sins both before and after our moment of salvation require Jesus' blood to cover them.

Condemnation is defined as the expression of very strong disapproval as well as the action of condemning someone to a punishment.[16] The Word tells us that Jesus did *not* come to condemn the world (John 12:47). He came to save it! There is no condemnation in Christ Jesus (Romans 8:1). When we are saved, we cannot do anything that makes God disapprove of who we are. He can disapprove of our idolatrous actions, but He still looks at us as His son or daughter and sees Jesus' blood covering us. He approves of us! He does not seek to punish us. Sin carries consequences, and God will allow those consequences in our lives to mold us to be more Christlike, but sin's punishment was carried out on the cross through Christ.

Satan wants us to run away from God when we mess up and presents thoughts that deceive us into thinking God will be mad at us and punish us. It's hard for us to see God as bigger than our sin. Satan shames us and whispers, "What's wrong with you?" We *feel* the condemnation of sin and shame. However, we need to cling to what we *know* God says.

Condemnation from Satan focuses on the problem and avoids the answer while pointing us to the things that serve as

Band-Aids. If we don't learn to trust God with our Band-Aids, we won't trust Him with healing our deepest wounds. Psalm 147:3 says that God heals the brokenhearted and binds up our wounds.

For the believer, shame is external — not internal. Remember, Satan throws shame on us like a cloak around our shoulders. This cloak can feel like a heavy weight of despair at times. Satan knows that if we walk around under the weight of his shame, we won't grab hold of and cling to the healing available for us because we will be too busy looking at our sin instead of how Jesus redeemed us from it.

Part of our emotional eating struggle is due to not allowing God to get into our pain and heal it. We've become quite the escape artists. When our pain is triggered, we escape into food and so many other things. Because we escape and make choices that devalue ourselves, Satan heaps a lot of shame on us from our traumas and our choices, simultaneously manipulating the truth about how God sees us. So eating becomes a form of self-punishment. We don't believe we are valuable or worth the effort of treating ourselves with respect, and since we feel shameful anyway, we continue the cycle of emotional eating.

Let's see how shame works as an internal trigger and becomes its own cycle that we can easily get stuck in.

SHAME

S

The "S" of shame is for Satan's schemes. Picture the bottom part of the S as a bowl.

Satan pulls from an ingredient list of other people's words, our own thoughts, and his lies from past experiences where we've fallen into temptation or been hurt and creates the perfect "condemnation recipe" that is specific to each of us. He waits for the perfect moment when the recipe is complete, and then he dumps the whole thing upside down into our hearts.

Satan is always working to shame us and create distance between us and God. He often uses our lack of intimacy with

God as the cracked door to get in and delay us from our purpose and healing so that we remain under the cloak of shame. Some signs to recognize are feelings of powerlessness against triggers, fear, embarrassment, and confusion.

As we learned with the three As of intentionality, if we don't analyze what's going on in our minds, annihilate Satan's lies, and appropriate Jesus' truth, this diabolical concoction will turn into belief systems that will be reflected in our actions.

H

The "H" of shame is for our hearts, where belief systems are solidified.

Out of the mouth, the heart speaks. Luke 6:45 says, "A good man brings good things out of the good stored up in his heart, and an evil man brings evil things out of the evil stored up in his heart. For the mouth speaks what the heart is full of." As a man thinks in his heart, so is he.

We can say the "right" things about ourselves to others — often hiding behind what we think we *should* say — but words are empty when spoken by someone who believes the opposite. If we believe Satan's lies and don't implement thought control, we adopt these lies into our belief systems. We begin to think of ourselves as Satan does, and it eventually shows up in our speech and actions. <callout> Our hearts believe what our minds leave unguarded.<callout> We agree with either God or Satan about who we are. Take a wild guess at which one is *for* you and which one is *against* you.

A

The "A" of shame is for actions — those of commission and omission.

These are actions we have taken, actions others have taken against us, and actions we and others should have taken but did not. Satan weaves all of these together into a cloak of shame.

We act out what we believe about ourselves, God, others, and our circumstances. By taking inventory of our actions, it's fairly easy to figure out what our belief systems are. Satan's strategy of keeping us in the stronghold of emotional eating is to highlight the actions of eating, exercising, dieting, etc. and keep us from looking at the messages we are believing.

We must shift our focus from our actions to the truth God wants to reveal to us about what's behind them. We need to start looking at our behavior as a window that allows us to see a deeper heart issue. The heart issue is the need for Jesus — not just for salvation, but for the power and strength that creates a life of freedom. If we don't intentionally shift this focus, our actions will create a negative space for Satan to fill our minds with more lies.

M

The "M" of shame is for the manipulated messages from Satan.

Satan sends us these manipulated messages mixed with our own thoughts, and he winds us up like a top that keeps spinning.

Messages from Satan will always be turned against us. We see that in those "I told you so" moments: "See, you don't have the strength to withstand temptation. See, they hurt you because you're not worth loving and being valued." His messages attach to everything we do and everything that is done to us. Once we believe him, we view God from his perspective. This manipulation also stops us from seeing ourselves and our sin from God's perspective, causing us to walk around under the weight of shame and low self-worth. We reach for food to hide our true and vulnerable selves from others and God.

Satan's lies cause a deficit in our heart, so we interact with God from a belief system that says He is holding out on us. We don't see God for who He really is — a good Father providing for and protecting us.

The truth is that we do not have strength on our own to withstand temptation. But Satan manipulates us into focusing on our lack of strength instead of the power we have been given by God to endure temptation and overcome it, as we read earlier in 1 Corinthians 10:13. God wants to set the record straight and remind us that a supernatural result of following Jesus is that we won't give into temptation if we only turn to Him.

E

The "E" of shame is for embarrassment.

Satan keeps the focus on us, and because of his manipulated messages, we become embarrassed of ourselves. Shame is always directed inward and makes *us* the ones to be embarrassed about; it attacks our identities. Shame will always cause us to be embarrassed about who we are. It attacks our self-worth and makes it hard to look at ourselves in the mirror. We hide from ourselves, self-sabotage, punish ourselves, and let others mistreat us. We continue devaluing ourselves because we believe our worth is based on what others think or what our actions say about us. We settle for what feels good in the moment because we don't believe our long-term success is worth fighting for. Then we walk around with a smile on our face, acting as if we are really OK. This embarrassment causes us to lose sight of grace. Satan then has us right where he wants us, with the focus yet again on our actions and ourselves.

I feel emotionally exhausted just writing about this cycle, and to know I've lived it for so long blows my mind. Aren't you exhausted, my friend?

This is a very real place many of us attempt to live in, yet we don't reach out for help. I wasn't able to overcome the strongholds in my life without the power of the Holy Spirit and the accountability and transparency of my friends and mentors. These people met my sins with truth spoken in love and tenderness—without judgment but with an urgency to return to the foot of the cross for the mercy and grace that is so readily available from Jesus.

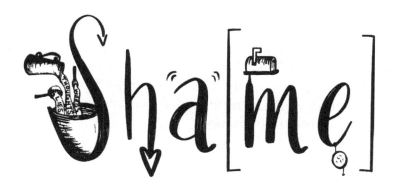

Do you see the cycle? There are two main loops to it. When we don't stop and implement intentional thought control against Satan's scheming lies at the "S," our hearts adopt the strongholds at the "H" that are all the false belief systems that result in us seeking shelter from reality in our actions at the "A." That's the first loop.

We then get bogged down with our actions and their consequences (or the pain of others' actions) at the "A," so our actions become self-fulfilling prophecies because we listen to Satan's manipulated messages at the "M." We then feel embarrassed at the "E" about who we are in this struggle and avoid looking at the "ME" of shame through God's eyes. That's the second loop.

This shame cycle operates as a self-sustaining machine consisting of the first loop of the S-H-A cycle of lies, beliefs, actions that pivots at the "A" into the second loop of the A-M-E cycle of actions, manipulation, and embarrassment. It's no wonder we feel hopeless.

Friend, shame is one of the most powerful weapons in Satan's arsenal. He lays it over us like a heavy cloak, and the feelings of overwhelm and hopelessness creep in and take up residence. We must intentionally throw off the cloak of shame and create an environment that makes shame unwelcome.

OVERCOMING SHAME

There is hope. His name is Jesus. He has given us tools and authority to take this shame from Satan and crush it. We saw how Satan uses *our actions* as the pivoting point for his two-loop system of shame. We must shift our focus to *Jesus' action* on the cross when He took the punishment and power of our sin away from us and gave us His freedom and power instead. Let's look at how we can fight against Satan's shame and stand firm against his condemnation.

S: *Spiritual Warfare*

When we mess up, we need to intentionally identify Satan's lies and replace them with God's truth. To fight against Satan's scheming, we must take part in spiritual warfare. We see in Ephesians 6:11 that we have been given armor and weapons of warfare when it says, "Put on the full armor of God, so that you can take your stand against the devil's schemes." When our thoughts devalue us, it's time to armor up.

We remind ourselves through the belt of truth that we will believe all of God's Word, which is the sword of the Spirit, and we claim what God says about us instead of believing what Satan says. We remind ourselves through the breastplate of righteousness that through Christ we have the ability to do what is right and pleasing to God. We will overcome because of Jesus' power in us. Through the helmet of salvation, we remind ourselves that we belong to Jesus, not Satan, and we lift up our shield of faith and trust that God's power and truth will crush the lies of Satan. We ready ourselves with our gospel shoes for the little things that lead us into temptation. Isaiah 59:17 adds the cloak of zeal into the mix, where we ask Jesus for a fresh dose of motivation and fervor to keep fighting. This cloak of zeal replaces the cloak of shame Satan throws around our shoulders.

We stop letting our feelings of embarrassment or frustration drive us away from God and make a choice to believe God is good, that He is *for* us, and that He wants to be gracious to us. The more we engage with Jesus through prayer, the more we learn to get up and run to Him quicker after the falls.

H: Humility

Humbling ourselves means we stop trying to act better than we are. We needed a Savior to pay the price for our sins as human beings. Why do we think that after salvation we will never sin again?

You might say, "I don't think that. I know we're human and imperfect. It's expected for us to sin. I know I'm not perfect." You know this intellectually, but remember, you *do* what you believe. When you sin and then fall into self-condemnation and pity (giving you permission to keep sinning instead of running to Jesus for grace and mercy), you reveal that you believe you could keep yourself from sinning in the first place.

As we fall more in love with Jesus, when we sin, we should feel heartbreak over our choice to sin against God. Sin should cause a deep sadness in our hearts, and when this sadness is present, it turns us toward God. However, if we are carrying a perfectionist belief system that we haven't owned up to yet, this is rooted in pride. Because of this lack of humility, we turn inward against ourselves and away from God after we sin instead of toward Him.

When we sin, we must humble ourselves and remember that this is the very reason Jesus chose to die. *We cannot overcome sin on our own.* We then ask God to reveal what's in our hearts just as David did in Psalm 139:23–24 (NLT): "Search me, O God, and know my heart; test me and know my anxious thoughts; point out anything in me that offends you, and lead me along the path of everlasting life." David made many stupid decisions, yet he was a man after God's heart. Despite his sins, he always humbled himself before God and repented. He believed the truth about who God was and how God saw him, and he didn't let his own sin distort those truths.

A: *Appropriation of Jesus' Righteousness*

We have been given the righteousness of Christ that lives within us through the Holy Spirit. Colossians 2:9–10 says, "For in Christ, all the fullness of the Deity lives in bodily form, and in Christ you have been brought to fullness." When we feel shame, it's easy to believe that we just can't get it together. Yet again, we find ourselves at the same place. Many things can trigger these self-defeating thoughts that make us want to stop fighting.

Something to remember when we are in this place of looking at our actions and allowing them to make us feel hopeless is that we are spending a lot of energy on self-defeating thoughts that lead to more self-sabotaging actions. This amount of energy, if redirected toward fighting against shame, could lead us to somewhere pretty great — more freedom.

I've said it before, and I'll say it again: Our choice button is not broken. We may not have chosen to get on the merry-go-round of Satan's shame, but once we realize we are there, we are definitely <u>choosing</u> to stay on it. Through Christ, this is within our power at any moment. We can reject the Devil's self-defeating lies and claim the righteousness given to us through the Holy Spirit. This power of righteousness is the ability to live in a way that is right in God's eyes. We *can*. We must stop agreeing with Satan that we *can't*. Last time I checked, Satan is still the loser against Jesus in the battle over sin and death. We are more than conquerors in Jesus.

M: *Memorization of God's Truth*

This is vital to our success. God gives us the blueprints on how not to sin against Him. Psalm 119:11 says, "I have hidden your word in my heart that I might not sin against you." From this verse, we see that we won't sin against God when we fight with His truths. The thing is, unfortunately, we don't always choose to fight. And all too often, when we do engage in the fight, it's on our own understanding or with a "can-do" attitude.

God calls Himself the Lion of Judah. He fights on our behalf. Satan is also called a lion, but one that is on the prowl seeking to devour us. When we fight with God's Word, we allow the lions to fight each other. I often think about this picture when I try to fight my own battles without leaning on God's truth. It would be like me going up against a lion by myself when I have the loyalty of a greater lion at my back waiting to fight for me. God's words fight for me. When I hide them in my heart and use them during times of temptation, I let the Lion of Judah demolish Satan's attack.

I have found a beautiful new strength where I can boldly tell Satan with authority that the junk of shame he's brought to the doorstep of my heart is absolutely no match for the Lion of Judah I have on the inside with me. I've gained so much ground because of knowing God's Word.

Let me show you how memorizing Scripture can help us overcome shame and keep us from sinning as often or in the same ways. This is how I fight once I've messed up: I follow David's example in the Psalms and talk to myself as a way to get more intentional. Sometimes we need to give ourselves solid, intentional pep talks. I call these my manifestos. I pray that this inspires you to carve out your own versions inspired by Scripture. Create three separate manifestos, one for each of the trigger, eating, and shame phases.

Trigger Phase Manifesto

Jenna! Enough. Put feelings in the backseat and command truth to get in the driver's seat. Take captive your thoughts (2 Corinthians 10:5) and make them obey God's truth. Quit negotiating with Satan and put your hope in the Lord, not your ability to overcome your circumstances (Psalm 43:5). Cling to what God has taught you (John 8:31–32), and don't run back to the stronghold of food, but instead find refuge in Him (Psalm 61:2–3).

Eating Phase Manifesto

You have been given weapons (Ephesians 6:11), so pick them up, fight against your enemy, and think on things that honor God (Philippians 4:8). Put the food down and keep it in its rightful place — as a created thing (Romans 1:25). Claim your authority over Satan (Luke 10:19) and press forward (Philippians 3:13–14). Do not go into shame over this because you have been given grace, not condemnation (Romans 8:1).

Shame Phase Manifesto

Your decision to sin hasn't changed how God sees you, but it's going to change how you see yourself if you let it. Jesus chose the cross knowing your sin. He bore your sin willingly out of love (1 Peter 2:24). He has set you free (Galatians 5:1), so get up and walk in that freedom. Don't rely on your understanding of it all (Proverbs 3:5–6); ask God to show you where you turned wrong (Psalm 139:23). This was no surprise to God. He gave you an out, but you missed it. Be more aware next time (1 Corinthians 10:13). Go to the throne of grace (Hebrews 4:16) and let Jesus be your hiding place (Psalm 119:114). Get up, forget what's behind, and press forward.

E: *Enthralling Beauty*

God is enthralled with our beauty. He tells us that we are beautiful and we have His attention. He wants us to honor Him because He wants to give us Himself. He made us intricately (Psalm 139). It doesn't matter what we look like or what we do. It doesn't change the fact that we have been created beautifully in God's eyes. I don't understand why we put so much power in the hands of other created beings to define what beauty looks like.

As the crown of God's creation, He not only calls us good but *beautiful*. In fact, as my amazing editor pointed out, God said His creation was "good" until He made mankind. Then He said it was "*very* good" (Genesis 1:31)! He waits to have compassion on us and calls us the apple of His eye. We are desired by God, and nothing about us embarrasses Him. He sent His Son to die and win us back—that's how much He wants a relationship with us. This is what God says about us: "Let the king be enthralled by your beauty; honor Him, for He is your Lord" (Psalm 45:11, NIV). We must remember that when we are in Christ, God looks at us and sees Jesus all over us. He can't help but approve of us!

We have so many tools at our fingertips through God's Word. When we armor up and fight shame head-on, we demolish the lies of Satan that keep us in the shame cycle. If we don't combat Satan's shame, our perspective will remain on ourselves. We will then settle into condemnation and begin to wallpaper the walls of our strongholds. This accelerates the emotional eating cycle, and next time we reach for food even faster.

Fighting shame requires that we accept God's grace. Galatians 5:1 reminds us that it is "for freedom that Christ has set us free. Stand firm, then, and do not let yourselves be burdened again by a yoke of slavery." When we claim that we have already been set free from the slavery of emotional eating, we decelerate the cycle by rejecting Satan's shame.

GOING DEEPER

1. God wants us to come to Him when we mess up! Hebrews 4:16 (BSB) tells us to "approach the throne of grace with confidence, so that we may receive mercy and find grace to help us in our time of need." How do you normally act once you've messed up?

2. Condemnation from Satan focuses on the problem and avoids the answer while pointing us to the things that serve as Band-Aids. If we don't learn to trust God with our Band-Aids, we won't trust Him with healing our deepest wounds. If we carry around the shame of messing up, we won't see healing.

SHAME:

S: What are the ingredients of your shame recipe?

H: What belief systems have solidified in your heart?

A: What actions is Satan using to weave your cloak of shame?

M: What are your "I told you so" statements from Satan?

E: What are the devaluing statements you tell yourself?

Step into a new way of interacting with shame, take back the power from Satan, and stand firm against his condemnation when you mess up.

OVERCOMING SHAME:

S: Remind yourself of this scripture: Ephesians 6:11.

> Action Step: Spiritually armor-up and pick up your weapons.

H: Remind yourself of this scripture: Psalm 139:23–24.

> Action Step: Humble yourself and ask God to reveal what you're believing in your heart.

A: Remind yourself of this scripture: Colossians 2:9–10.

> Action Step: Act in a new way from the power of the Holy Spirit within you.

M: Remind yourself of this scripture: Psalm 119:11.

> Action Step: Memorize verses that help you stand firm.

E: Remind yourself of this scripture: Psalm 45:11.

> Action Step: Remind yourself daily that God is enthralled with your beauty.

Write your own manifestos:

> **Trigger Phase**
>
> **Eating Phase**
>
> **Shame Phase**

OWNING TRUTH

- Satan causes us to feel embarrassed about ourselves and attacks our worth and identity, but our responsibility as believers is to stand firm and engage in spiritual warfare.

- Satan forces our focus onto our actions instead of deeper heart issues. Fighting his shame requires us to accept God's grace. To reject Satan's shame is to claim our freedom in Jesus.

- Humbling ourselves before God, accepting His grace and mercy, and appropriating the righteousness of God within us through the Holy Spirit help us to choose differently and stay out of the shame cycle.

PART THREE:

End Emotional Eating

CHAPTER 8

Freedom Has Called My Name

I love war movies. The valor of the warriors who bravely fight for their cause and their loved ones moves something deep within me. It resonates with the message of Jesus as our mighty warrior, fighting for His cause and for His loved ones. I love the part in the movies where the warriors push through the wall of numerous enemy soldiers, destroying their stronghold and demolishing their weapons.

God is tenacious in bringing us to this point where we fight to take our freedom back and seek our hearts' fulfillment in Him instead of food. When we use His Word, it pushes through the wall of lies Satan has fed us—the stronghold of idolatry.

As much as I love the victory and valor in these movies, I can't deny a very real consequence of war: death. War is a serious business. We are in the middle of a spiritual battle whether we accept it or not. The reality is no matter how stubbornly we hide behind our strong-walled fortresses of faulty belief systems, there are still very real consequences of staying within a stronghold once we have been shown the exit. There is hope in this battle, however, because Jesus has not only called us to be warriors, but He has equipped us for this battle.

THE POWER OF A STRONGHOLD

God's Word says in 2 Corinthians 10:3-4, "For though we live in the world, we do not wage war as the world does. The weapons we fight with are not the weapons of the world. On the contrary, they have divine power to demolish strongholds." The Greek word for stronghold in this verse is *ochuróma*. It comes from the root word *oxyroō*, which means "to fortify." Ochuróma is used when describing a fortified military stronghold, a strong-walled fortress.[17] In the verse above, Paul uses this picture of a stronghold to help the reader better understand that a false argument — what we are believing — can be a shelter, or a "safe place," to escape reality.

This is a vital concept — God is revealing here that a stronghold of emotional eating is a false belief system in which we attempt to escape reality and seek out the shelter we believe food offers. Once we are enmeshed in this false belief system, we go into denial about the real consequences of sin. Turning to God for our fulfillment means we can't continue to hold onto false belief systems.

This is where our struggle gets a little harder. We must make the decision to let go of the faulty thinking patterns we escape into. We tend to wait until we *feel* ready to do so, but if we wait for our feelings to lead us to deny selfish desires and follow God's truth, we will wait forever. We must kick feelings out of the driver's seat and put God's truth in place and make a choice to believe God's Word. When we do this, we find ourselves on the path of denying self and walking in freedom. Do we do it perfectly? No. Do we do it more and more consistently? Yes. Take a few moments and ask God to reveal what your faulty belief systems are about food, yourself, circumstances, and the people in your life that keep you hiding behind your strong-walled fortress of emotional eating.

Let's talk about the foundational faulty belief system that Satan uses to keep us within our strongholds. It goes way back to before Jesus walked on this earth. God gave laws to Moses and the Israelites that were meant to highlight their inability to remain in good standing with Him on their own merits. Chosen priests were to make yearly animal sacrifices at the tabernacle to atone (make amends for) their sins and the sins of the people. This put them in good standing with God, but only temporarily.

The laws, when kept, helped people remain in a right relationship with God until it was time to make another sacrifice. Because these animal sacrifices were not enough to pay for the eternal aspect of sin and death, the priests had to keep sacrificing and seeking atonement for their sins every year.

Fast forward to when Jesus became the final and perfect blood sacrifice to atone for all sin. He won the victory by providing payment for sin and death for all eternity. He freed us from the need to continually sacrifice animals and follow laws to stay in good standing with God. Once we enter into a personal relationship with Jesus by faith through accepting God's gift of grace, we are freed from the punishment of sin and our sins are forgiven. Jesus' blood is what saves us—not anything we did or could do.

But Satan would have us believe otherwise. Sadly, so many people think that the way to gain God's approval and an eternity in Heaven is through legalistic rule-following. This is the foundational faulty belief system Satan uses. We can never be "good enough" to be right with God. When we sin against a law (for example, emotional eating/idolatry), we falsely believe we've been sent to the end of God's "approval line." We feel guilty (another false belief system) and then run to what we believe can help us escape the reality of our sin. In our case, we run to food. We hide from God just as Eve and Adam hid in the garden.

THE POWER OF GRACE

Ephesians 2:8 says, "For it is by grace you have been saved, through faith—and this is not from yourselves, it is the gift of

God." The Greek word for this grace is *xaris*, meaning that God freely extends Himself and His favor.[18] He reaches out to us and leans in to hear the prayers of His people because His character is to bless and be near those He loves and who love Him. Grace came on the scene through Jesus Christ. Romans 5:2 shows more of God's tenacious grace — through believing God, we are made righteous, and we can stand in grace because we stand *in* Christ.

What does "standing in" really mean? Have you ever gone swimming in the ocean? When you're in the ocean and the waves crash over you, you feel, taste, and smell like the ocean. There is no way around it. Christ's blood washes our sins away and His grace crashes over us like ocean waves. It's important to stay in the "ocean" of His sustaining grace to taste, feel, and smell like Christ. We can spend a lot of time at the beach and have full access to the ocean without ever jumping in.

It's time to jump in. Please don't sit at the shoreline, my friend. We have access to God because Jesus declared us righteous when we placed our faith in Him and began a relationship with Him. Being righteous means we are in good standing with God and have been given the power and ability to do what is right in God's eyes. Romans 4:3 tells us we were made righteous because of our faith in Christ and believing Him. We must ask ourselves if we are going to believe God fully or if we will hold a buffet-style belief system — taking only what we want and leaving the rest. We need to believe all of His words if we are going to believe any.

This gift of God's tenacious grace was offered to us when we were at our worst, as it tells us in Romans 5:8 (ESV), "But God shows his love for us in that while we were still sinners, Christ died for us." If God extended grace to us before salvation, why do we think God wouldn't extend it after we have been adopted as sons and daughters through salvation?

We are to cling boldly to the truth that Satan does not have power over us because we are submerged in the righteousness of Christ. Grace gives us the power to fight back!

We have been saved, and when we act like it, according to Romans 6:22 (ESV), we bear fruit. The Greek word for this fruit is *karpos*, meaning a figurative harvest or profit—everything done in partnership with Christ.[19] The Lord empowers us in this life to create something of eternal worth. Jesus' saving and sustaining grace is the exit strategy when we're locked in a stronghold.

THE PARADOX OF GRACE AND LAW

Now that we understand that grace is necessary to shut down the reign of sin in our strongholds, we should be good to go, right? I wish! But no, we humans like to complicate the truths of God. We often fearfully and stubbornly withhold our hearts' surrender from God and forfeit the intimacy of truly knowing and being known by Him. The Christian walk consists of a continual choosing between flesh and Spirit. It's a lifelong process that requires commitment. Paul understood this well and wrote about the paradox of grace versus sin in Romans 6:12–23.

How does the law of grace overcome the law of sin and death? It's something like the law of motion and its principle of lift and thrust overcoming the law of gravity. One law is higher and supersedes the other law. Planes fly because of the principles of lift and thrust that supersede gravity, but they only remain in flight with a pilot and an intentional system that puts boundaries in place. We are to live and walk in the freedom that Christ's righteousness has given us. Even under the law of grace, which supersedes the law of sin and death, we still need to follow God's commands as boundaries and parameters to keep us from crashing.

What happens when we let sin reign in us? The same thing that would happen if a plane flew with no boundaries or parameters, no checks or balances—it would crash! Satan loves to lie about freedom. We tend to believe that the freedom of eating how and when we want is something we can control, but like the plane, we crash and burn every time. When we are "free" from our allegiance to righteousness and give in to idolatry, the fruit of our actions is shame and regret. In the moment, we believe that eating what we want equates to freedom, but we are deceived into believing we can control the consequences of our actions.

This is why we cannot use grace as permission to sin. When we engage in the idolatry of emotional eating, we offer parts of our bodies to sin. This gives Satan weapons of unrighteousness to wield against us, distorting the truth that our sin doesn't change God's acceptance of and love for us. We stay in a lifestyle of shameful choices because of this distortion, and we are left with the consequences sin brings.

When we misuse our freedom, we build strongholds. Grace abounds for us throughout this process, but personally, I don't want the bad fruit of idolatry even if there is more grace waiting. I'll stick with going straight to grace, which will help me not to make idolatrous choices to begin with.

Because of our faith in Christ, we are now dead to sin (Romans 6:1–11). This means our debt has been paid, and death is no longer looking for us to pay up. We are also made alive in Christ, which means we have been placed back in good standing with God. Those of us who are alive in Christ are to offer ourselves to God (every part of ourselves) as weapons for righteousness against Satan. This corrects Satan's distortion and reminds him that, because we have been accepted by Christ, we don't have to remain under shame. Yes, we still stumble and sin, but we can continue walking in freedom rather than getting bogged down in shame.

THE POWER OF FREEDOM

If we belong to Christ, we are no longer condemned. Our status is that of a beloved child, not a guilty and condemned sinner. A rich woman acting like a poor woman living on the streets doesn't make her poor, but it makes her experience a life of poverty and all the hardship that comes with it. That may seem like a ridiculous scenario, but haven't we all done this? How often do we let our failures keep us feeling guilty (which leads to more failure), allowing our sin to rule over us long after the sinful act? We are rich beyond belief in Christ's power, yet we choose to live in the gutter.

In contrast, when we act as though we've been justified, sin will not rule over us. Romans 6:14 says, "For sin will not rule over you, because you are not under law, but under grace." The Greek word for sin here is *hamartia*, meaning the brand of sin that emphasizes its self-originated, self-empowered nature; it is something not originated or empowered by God.[20] The Greek word for rule is *kurieuó*, meaning to have authority, to exercise rights over one's own property as an owner with full dominion or lordship over this jurisdiction.[21] When we walk around beating ourselves up and believing we're guilty and condemned because we messed up yet again, we are deceived in thinking we are still under death's jurisdiction. When we refuse to believe God's truth about our redeemed status, this is the brand of sin where we exercise "rights" over our own body.

We're reminded in 1 Corinthians 6:20 that we were bought with the blood of Christ, which is where grace comes from, and therefore exercising our "rights" over our own body is in direct contradiction to God's Word. We choose to sin, then we become our own judge and condemn ourselves as guilty. This causes us to pull away and hide from God. We come to our own rescue by turning to something we believe we can control: food. We need to quit living a fairytale of our own making where we are the damsels in distress as well as the knights in shining armor. We cannot need help and help ourselves at the same time.

This self-sustaining brand of sin won't rule over us when we walk in the freedom of grace. God's Word clearly tells us we are under God's jurisdiction. When we believe this truth, we will get up quickly after we mess up, we'll dust ourselves off, and we'll thank God for His Lordship of grace over us. We won't carry around the baggage of sin, and we'll become less enslaved to it. Are there still consequences to sin? Yes, but we don't have to stay spiritually and emotionally stuck because of it.

We, as humans, owed a death debt. Jesus' righteousness paid that debt, and He gave us His strength and righteousness. We are being called to honor God by acting like rich women who have been given a gift of grace-filled righteousness. We need to quit acting like poor women escaping the reality of our sin and taking "refuge" in Satan's lies. When we have been saved, by grace through faith, we are to serve God — not self. We can achieve this when God is in "the God seat."

Have you had a defining moment where you willingly entered into a relationship with Jesus Christ and placed Him on the throne of your heart and life? Have you accepted His gift of grace and through faith believed He is the only One who can forgive your sins and invite you to spend eternity in Heaven with Him? If you have not had this moment, please take this time to connect with Jesus as your Savior. It takes a choice, your choice to believe God's Word that says He loves you so much He provided His Son, Jesus, to take your place on spiritual death row. He says that it is by His grace that you can be saved, through faith; there's nothing you can do or need to do other than accept the gift of salvation through Jesus.

Once you make this choice, you'll receive Jesus' Holy Spirit, who will walk with you and empower you to live in freedom. He waits eagerly to show you this grace. Isaiah 30:18 (NASB) — the Tenacious Grace theme verse — says,

> Therefore, the Lord longs to be gracious to you,
> And therefore He waits on high to have compassion on you.
> For the Lord is a God of justice;
> How blessed are all those who long for Him.

How will you respond?

If you have made this decision, please reach out to a leader at your church or a friend who is a Christ follower to let them know. You may also contact me, as I would love to help you along the way and get you connected to someone who can encourage and support you. My contact information is in the back of this book.

Your salvation is the foundation you'll need to stand firm on when Satan's attacks come your way. You'll learn to stand firm by paying attention to what does and doesn't work during the times of testing and training your faith. It all starts with fighting with the right weapons.

GOING DEEPER

1. When we choose not to believe God's truth about our redeemed status, we choose the brand of sin where we exercise "rights" over our own body. We then we become our own judge and condemn ourselves as guilty. This causes us to pull away and hide from God. We come to our own rescue by turning to something we believe we can control: food. What does your cycle of exercising "rights" over your own body look like?

2. What lies from Satan make you feel that your ability to accept grace and not turn to food isn't as strong as your ability to fall under the temptation of emotional eating?

3. Revisit the moments where you surrendered your life to Christ and were saved by accepting His gift of grace.

OWNING TRUTH

- A rich woman acting like a poor woman living on the streets doesn't make her poor, but it makes her experience a life of poverty and all the hardship that comes with it.

- We are being called to honor God by acting like rich women who have been given a gift of grace-filled righteousness. We need to quit acting like poor women escaping the reality of our sin and taking "refuge" in Satan's lies.

- It's time we quit living a fairytale of our own making where we are the damsels in distress as well as the knights in shining armor. We cannot need help and help ourselves at the same time.

CHAPTER 9

I Am Stronger Than I Think

Learning how to love God through obedience is a battle. At times, the spiritual struggle can feel like a never-ending, days-on-end fight to the death—one that ebbs and flows with small victories and small defeats.

At times, you will curl up in a ball and weep because of the inner battle. Exhaustion will come over you, and you'll want to crumble under the reality that if you choose to grow stagnant, you will usher in more pain and destruction from the enemy. So you keep fighting.

Other times, you will grin from ear to ear because of the ground you've gained fighting against the enemy's attacks and walking toward truth. You'll grow in intimacy and trust as you come closer to Jesus.

Still other times, you'll rebelliously choose to go back to the stronghold you thought you had destroyed.

We have learned about the emotional eating cycle and how triggers lead to emotional eating, followed by shame, which loops us back into more triggers, and we're off to the races again. In this chapter, we will study how we can gain even more ground and move forward in leaps instead of baby steps along the way. We will study the weapons of warfare God has given us to demolish our strongholds for good.

I can confidently say that no soldier would choose to go onto the battlefield without their weapons or battle gear. We are in a spiritual battle, yet many days we wake up and go into our day without putting on armor or using our weapons. We get beaten down because we aren't engaging in the battle — we're getting swept up in it.

If we want to walk in freedom from our strongholds, we must use the weapons God has given us in Ephesians 6:10–18. Isn't it time we learned how to fight and warrior-up when those attacks from Satan come our way?

STAND YOUR GROUND

This is God's command to us:

> Finally, be strong in the Lord and in his mighty power. Put on the *full* armor of God, so that you can take your stand against the devil's schemes. For our struggle is not against flesh and blood, but against the rulers, against the authorities, against the powers of this dark world and against the spiritual forces of evil in the heavenly realms. Therefore, put on the *full* armor of God, so that when the day of evil comes, you may be able to stand your ground, and after you have done everything, to stand. Stand firm then, with the *belt of truth* buckled around your waist, with the *breastplate of righteousness* in place, and with your feet fitted with the readiness that comes from the *gospel of peace*. In addition to all this, take up the *shield of faith*, with which you can extinguish all the flaming arrows of the evil one. Take the *helmet of salvation* and the *sword of the Spirit*, which is the word of God.

And *pray* in the Spirit on all occasions with all kinds of prayers and requests. With this in mind, be alert and always keep on praying for all the Lord's people [emphasis added].

Whenever words like "finally" or "therefore" show up in Scripture, it's important to look at what came before those verses. If we look at the beginning of Chapter 6, Paul is instructing Christians on how to have God-honoring households. He is talking about consistency in Christian living and how it hinges on being strong in the Lord and His mighty power. He then proceeds to tell Christians how to be triumphant under attack.

Something to note is that Paul was writing this letter to the church at Ephesus while he was imprisoned in Rome. The fact that he writes this from a prison cell is an inspiration for Christians to apply the same truths he practiced. Someone whose spirit is broken due to circumstances doesn't write letters that impact lives thousands of years later—Paul practiced what he preached. Peace and contentment accompanied him in the circumstances to which God called him. He fought the good fight, and he fought well. I'm sure he had depressing days and hard times, but he put the principles of spiritual warfare into practice, and we have his example to prove their effectiveness.

I'll highlight a few noteworthy points before getting into the specific weapons. We see Paul tells us to put on the full armor of God twice before he says what the pieces of armor are. He wanted to make sure we understood his point about the *full* armor, not just a piece here and there. To stand against the Devil's schemes, we need every bit of spiritual protection.

Paul uses active verbs and instructs us to either "stand against" or "stand firm" four times. We have a choice each time we are tempted to emotionally eat. Remember that choice button? Well, it isn't broken—after all, we choose to put on our self-made armor, don't we? Some of our defenses may look like denial, isolation, anger, self-righteousness, justification, control, or planning for the next food fix. In the face of dealing with our emotions, these are only a handful of the defense mechanisms that make up the whole getup of self-sufficient idolatry. Take a few moments and ask the Lord to identify the armor you're putting on instead of His armor.

You must realize this struggle isn't against flesh and blood. It is not with the person who offended or wounded you. It's not with your body or the people you compare yourself to. Yes, you interact with those and can get tripped up, but your struggle is against the spiritual forces of evil, including Satan and the demons who serve him. And you can defeat these forces! The Lord says you have been given authority to "tread on snakes and scorpions, and over all the power of the enemy. Nothing will harm you" (Luke 10:19, BSB).

Paul tells us to put on the armor so that when the day of evil comes, we can stand firm. He says *when*, not *if*. If you're not expecting a spiritual attack, you have unrealistic expectations. Christians would be much greater warriors if they were always on guard. Instead, spiritual warfare comes as a surprise to many believers. This is where Satan gains ground — through sneak attacks against unprepared warriors.

> This is where Satan gains ground — through sneak attacks against unprepared warriors.

ARMORED UP

Paul, a prisoner, would have had plenty of time to study a Roman soldier's armor. He uses the pieces of armor as metaphors, connecting them to the spiritual truth of our position in Christ.

I get so excited talking about our weapons of warfare and the armor God gives us because, secretly, I want to be Wonder Woman and have out-of-this-world powers to dominate my enemies. I picture myself fearlessly standing against the enemy forces as I fight for freedom from oppression. God reminds me that in Him, I am a wonder woman, and I do have spiritual power to tear down Satan and his lies.

Friend, we have weapons and power beyond our understanding to fight for the freedom already obtained for us by Jesus.

Belt of Truth

Called the *cingulum* or *balteus* in Roman times, the belt held a scabbard, which kept the sword in place. Without the belt, the soldier wouldn't have a way to keep his sword ready when needed. The belt of truth allows us to use the sword of the Spirit, God's Word.

I think the belt is listed first because if we don't believe that God's Word is true, we won't use the remaining armor and weapons. How often do we try to tackle the emotional and spiritual battle pushing us toward food without first buckling God's truth in place? Too often. Jesus modeled how to fight spiritual warfare when He was tempted in the wilderness in Matthew 4. He believed God's Word was true, and when He was tempted, He used Scripture every time to fight back. He stood firm.

Peter tells us in 1 Peter 5:8 (Holman Christian Standard Bible) to "Be serious! Be alert! Your adversary the Devil is prowling around like a roaring lion, looking for anyone he can devour." Imagine a roaring lion circling you, waiting to devour you. It would be understandable to cower in fear and give in to the demands of this lion—if you didn't remember the truth that God, the Lion of Judah, is fighting for you.

To help you better understand this concept, let me share how cowering to the demands of the lion looked for me. I mistakenly placed the power to define my worth in men's hands. Whenever I was in a situation where a guy was pursuing me romantically, I listened to the lies of the roaring, circling lion. Satan told me I was valuable only if I had a relationship to define me. Because I wrongly believed that a man could determine my worth, I felt I couldn't turn down any relationship. I gave in to the demands of Satan's lies and entered into unhealthy attachments that left my heart shattered many times over.

Here is the truth, my friend. Psalm 17:13 (ESV) says, "Arise, O Lord! Confront him, subdue him! Deliver my soul from the wicked by your sword." I love this psalm because it shows that God will fight for us and be our refuge. He strengthens us and then invites us to join Him in the battle. God fought for me and brought me out of those wrong belief systems with His truth, and over time, the shattered pieces of my heart were mended. I now stand strong against the lies of the enemy. Today, I have no problem turning down a relationship that won't have Christ at its center. In Romans 8:37, Paul reminds us that we are more than conquerors through Jesus. We are warriors fighting an enemy, but we have the guarantee of victory — we need only seize it.

Breastplate of Righteousness

In ancient battles, protecting one's vital organs was of the utmost importance. If a soldier's lungs were punctured, he would no longer be able to breathe, much less fight — that's why soldiers wore breastplates. When we have our breastplate in place, we breathe in the righteousness of Christ and breathe out a life full of choices that honor God. Righteousness means we have been approved of and given the ability to do what is right in God's eyes. Through grace, Christ has extended Himself to us; therefore, the righteousness of Christ was placed in us (Romans 3:26). We need to remember we have full access to His ability to choose rightly.

In Jeremiah 17:9, we learned how our hearts can deceive us, and Proverbs 4:23 says we are to protect our hearts with all vigilance. We can easily be led astray when following the path our hearts set before us. Instead, we must yield to the power of Christ within us. When we put on the breastplate of righteousness, it guards us against our hearts, protects our hearts from the unhealthy influence of others, and reminds us that we can succeed through the righteousness given to us by Christ — not our own strength.

When I experience moments of temptation to emotionally eat, I sometimes place my hand on my chest to remind myself that my heart is protected by Jesus' ability to choose Him and not food. When we don't act as though we have Jesus' righteousness flowing through our spiritual veins, we leave ourselves open to damaging attacks. How many of our hearts have been shredded because of the unrighteous choices we have made?

Gospel of Peace Shoes

Our next piece of armor is our spiritual shoes. Ephesians tells us to have our feet fitted with the readiness that comes from the gospel of peace.

When I was young, the house I lived in had a large backyard that was filled with the best trees, perfect for climbing, and plenty of room to run. I loved to walk around barefoot when I was a kid (and still do), but one of the things I remember most about that yard was how I couldn't run barefoot as much as I wanted because of the "gumballs" (seed capsules of the sweetgum tree) that had fallen to the ground. I would take off running through the grass — then my foot would slam down on a spiky gumball that would stop me dead in my tracks and send me limping back to the house. I had a choice: I could stay in the house, or I could put on shoes that would protect against those prickly little suckers and get back outside and run. I chose the shoes. My shoes helped me run freely, without fear.

Satan tends to leave the big artillery for our vital spiritual organs, our minds and hearts, but he won't hesitate to throw out gumball-sized attacks to slow us down so we walk cautiously instead of running boldly. Most often, we emotionally eat because of the stress that results from all the gumballs of life in our path (computer glitches, busy schedules, long lines, endless errands, housework, etc.). We must be prepared by knowing the *truth* so we can choose *righteously* and put on our "ready to handle the little things" shoes to stand firm and run into the fight.

As we run onto this battlefield, another aspect of our spiritual shoes is that we carry with us the gospel of peace. There is no peace to be found on a battlefield; we must bring it with us. To have peace in our lives, we remind ourselves that we carry the peace that comes from Christ. John 14:25–27 tells us that Jesus gives us peace in the form of the Holy Spirit. When we belong to Christ, we are walking vessels of peace. Even when the battle rages around us, we can intentionally tap into the peace that comes from the Holy Spirit.

Shield of Faith

We have been given a shield of faith that can extinguish all the flaming arrows of the evil one. The Roman shield was called the *scutum*. It was very large—some types were almost three and a half feet high—and in the shape of a curved rectangle.

The shield was a defensive weapon, but at its center was a large metal knob called a *boss* that soldiers used to bash their opponents. I just love the fact that this extra piece on the shield is called a *boss* because when we use this weapon in battle against Satan, we can show him who's boss with the authority given to us by God. The boss allows us to go on the offensive and shove Satan out of our faces so that we can pull out our sword of the Spirit and cut him down with truth.

Can you see it? Can you see the close combat where we cut down all of the Devil's lies? All of his lies are fiery darts meant to engulf us in spiritual flames. When we use the shield, we have the promise that it will extinguish those lies. Our faith renders Satan powerless.

Up until now, we have only seen pieces of armor that we can wear. Once we put them on, they stay until we take them off. When we believe Satan's lies and act out of an idolatrous heart, we take off the belt of truth that tells us we are guaranteed the victory and that food doesn't fulfill our hearts. We take off the breastplate of righteousness that reminds us we have the power to choose the right way and say no to the food when we aren't physically hungry. We also take off the shoes of the gospel of peace that remind us we have peace within us through the Holy Spirit and can run boldly. There is a natural consequence when we take off these pieces of armor: we're going to feel the pain of Satan's attacks. It's so important not only to put on these pieces daily but also to be intentional in not removing them.

Our shield of faith is something we must carry with us and use over and over again. We make a choice to believe God and use our weapons in the battle. Faith is described in Hebrews 11:1 (ESV) as the "assurance of things hoped for, the conviction of things not seen." With the shield, we can do incredible damage and gain ground in our fight against idolatry and Satan's attacks.

Helmet of Salvation

The helmet protects the brain, another vital organ. Many of our battles start in our minds. God tells us to be transformed by the renewing of our minds. He instructs us to take our thoughts captive, and since emotions start in the mind, we must be on guard. We have been given the mind of Christ just as we've been given His power. Aligning our mind with His, we can operate as He wants us to. We can think differently because of the Holy Spirit in us. To do so, we must implement thought control and practice intentionality and accountability.

We have the helmet of salvation to remind us we have been redeemed by the blood of Christ. This redemption is what gives us power from the Holy Spirit. The biggest benefit of being saved and belonging to Christ is that we know the God of the universe fights for us and protects us. Romans 8:31 (HCSB) says, "What then are we to say about these things? If God is for us, who is against us?" Will the journey and battle be easy? No. Will we be protected and provided for through the process? Yes.

If we fight out in the open on our own strength, we will end up bloody and bruised. Instead, we can fight in the shadow of God's protective wing as it tells us in Psalm 91:4. We engage in the battle, but only with the circumstances, thoughts, and feelings that have passed through God's warrior hands first.

Sword of the Spirit

The sword in Roman times was called a *gladius*. It had a short blade with two sharpened edges and was so powerful that it could cut through metal. The sword of the Spirit is such a powerful weapon that God says in Hebrews 4:12 (HCSB) it is "living and effective and sharper than any double-edged sword, penetrating as far as the separation of soul and spirit, joints and marrow. It is able to judge the ideas and thoughts of the heart."

Scripture is our most effective weapon against Satan's attacks. To escape his clutches, we must replace his lies with truth. So many times, we want to just "stop thinking" certain things. We can't ignore the lies because Satan will keep coming with more of them. We need to practice *replacing* lies with truth, not just trying to *stop* thinking them. If we don't know what God's Word says about idolatry, our worth, and other matters of life and godliness, we will get triggered and fall into negotiations with the enemy.

Like the shield of faith, the sword of the Spirit is used for close combat. This is where it gets personal. Some of Satan's most personal attacks are against our worth, identity, and position in Christ. Too many times, we go up against Satan without knowing what scriptures to use, but when we memorize verses and fight with them, they pack a whole lot of punch.

Cloak of Zeal

This is a piece of armor that tends to be overlooked. Isaiah 59:17 (HCSB) says, "He put on righteousness like a breastplate, and a helmet of salvation on His head; He put on garments of vengeance for clothing, and He wrapped Himself in zeal as in a cloak." In Roman times, cloaks protected people against the cold and served as makeshift beds and protection from the rain. They had natural oils in the fabric that made them almost waterproof. A cold, wet, and tired soldier won't perform at optimal strength and endurance.

Zeal is defined as "having great energy or enthusiasm in pursuit of a cause or an objective."[22] When we are zealously following Christ, we will value the things that help us fight at optimal strength and with great fervor. This can be our physical health (regular sleep, healthy diet, exercise, and rest), spiritual and emotional rejuvenation, soul care, etc. Zeal is the fuel of our internal passion for following Christ.

Have you lost your zeal to do God's work? To keep pressing forward toward more freedom? To put the truth you've learned through this journey into practice? To follow Christ's example and stay in the battle? Please pray for God to wrap you daily in a cloak of zeal. Ask Him to fuel a fire so strong within your spirit that your energy and enthusiasm reflect a new commitment to pursue freedom from idolatry/emotional eating. Stay faithful in your prayers for this. Your renewed mindset will lead your emotions to get in line.

Prayer

Paul completes his list of armor with the admonishment to "pray in the Spirit on all occasions with all kinds of prayers and requests." Have you ever thought that prayer—communication with God—could be a vital part of overcoming your strongholds and claiming the victory in spiritual warfare?

Imagine going into battle without any way to communicate with your commander. In ancient warfare, soldiers had to send messages by way of horns, trumpets, and signals. Military technology has come a long way, but regardless of *how* warriors stay in contact, they *must* do so. In order to plot attacks and defenses against the enemy, soldiers have to communicate with each other—and with their commander. If they don't, they are left to guess where the enemy forces are, how powerful their weapons are, how or when they'll attack, and whether or not any reinforcements are on the way.

Prayer is a huge advantage against our enemy. Praying for others and ourselves as well as asking others to pray for us keeps us connected and strengthened. Too many times, we scramble to stay in the fight and clumsily fling our weapons around without any real direction because we aren't communicating with our Commander. We walk through our days guessing at what is really going on and reacting with self-protective measures.

This ushers in a state of spiritual and emotional confusion that leads straight to emotional eating. This is where prayer must be a vital part of our daily lives.

Words hold great power. The words that are exchanged between you and God during prayer will have a powerful impact on your life. Prayer is a purposeful repositioning of our hearts and minds back under the lordship of Christ — our Commander for the glory of God through the power of the Holy Spirit. It places us in communication with the One who not only knows our enemy well but has already defeated him. It's important to understand the power our words hold — with ourselves and with God.

God chose to speak the world into existence instead of forming it with His hands as He did humans. We learn two things from this truth: The words we speak to ourselves have power as we use them to either agree with God or agree with Satan, and God is intimately involved with us in a hands-on way. God not only wants you to communicate with Him through prayer, but He also wants to walk through this battle with you. Prayer brings you into a closer relationship with Him and activates the power of the words shared between you.

THE MODEL WARRIOR

When Jesus was tempted to worship Satan (Matthew 4:8–10), He chose to worship God alone. Jesus was ready for Satan because He wore His spiritual shoes: the readiness that comes from the gospel of peace. He believed God's commands to be true because He wore His helmet of salvation (He knew His position as God's Son). He righteously chose to engage in the fight instead of cowering because He wore His breastplate of righteousness. Jesus took up His shield of faith, showed Satan who was boss, and shoved him back with the words "go away," and then had the faith to use His sword of the Spirit and repeat God's words when saying "worship the lord your God and serve only Him" (Matthew 4:10 CEV). Jesus wore His cloak of zeal as He pursued His Father's will for His life and diligently sought a relationship with God. He was in communication with His Father and the Spirit through prayer while fasting 40 days and nights in the wilderness.

> Then Jesus told him, "Go away, Satan! For it is written:
>   Worship the Lord your God,
>   and serve only Him."
> Then the Devil left Him, and immediately angels came and began to serve Him."
>
> —Matthew 4:10–11 (HCSB)

I'm so thankful we have this warrior fighting on our behalf. Jeremiah 20:11 (ESV) says, "But the Lord is with me as a dread warrior; therefore my persecutors will stumble; they will not overcome me. They will be greatly shamed, for they will not succeed. Their eternal dishonor will never be forgotten." On this spiritual battlefield, our persecutors are Satan and his army. When we keep our armor on, use our weapons, and follow Jesus into battle, we will have the victory. The reprieve and reward come *after* we've engaged in the battle.

GOING DEEPER

1. What pieces of your own armor have you chosen to put on instead of God's?

2. Where do you look for peace other than Christ?

3. What truths from God's Word do you use to counteract Satan's lies?

Take a minute and list the people and circumstances you want to be more specific in praying about. Then write out a prayer asking God to renew your zeal and rekindle your energy and enthusiasm in pursuit of freedom from emotional eating.

OWNING TRUTH

*   We are reminded through our breastplate of righteousness that we can easily be led astray when following our heart. Instead of following our feelings, we must yield to the power of Christ within us that gives us the ability to choose rightly.

*   When we use the shield of faith, we have the promise that it will extinguish the lies that drive us to emotional eating. Our faith renders Satan powerless.

*   Prayer is a purposeful repositioning of our hearts and minds back under the lordship of Christ for the glory of God through the power of the Holy Spirit.

CHAPTER 10

The Power of Support Systems

At this point, hopefully, you've done the work it takes to define your different relationships with different foods, understand the idolatry of emotional eating, discern between the different types of hunger, identify the triggers and shame surrounding your eating, and learn how God tenaciously gives you the freedom to fight with spiritual weapons and overcome with victory.

UNDERSTANDING ACCOUNTABILITY

How many times have we tried to go it alone? How is that working for us? When we choose to fight the battle of overcoming emotional eating alone, we choose to fail. The beauty of having accountability in our lives is that it provides a place for us to be honest and take responsibility for our actions along the way. Being accountable means you are required or expected to justify your actions or decisions; it's being responsible.[23]

As Christians, we will stand in front of Holy God on judgment day and give an account for our actions. Romans 14:11–12 says, "It is written: 'As surely as I live,' says the LORD, 'every knee will bow before me; every tongue will acknowledge God.' So then, each of us will give an account of ourselves to God." When that day comes, what will your account look like? When God asks why you chose to worship food instead of Him, what will your justification be for your choices?

Accountability to God is lived out through interacting with other members of the body of Christ so that we hold one another accountable. 1 Corinthians 12:12, 27 (ESV) says, "For just as the body is one and has many members, and all the members of the body, though many, are one body, so it is with Christ. . . . Now you are the body of Christ and individually members of it." Ecclesiastes 4:12 tells us there is power in numbers. Ephesians 5:21 says, "Submit to one another out of reverence for Christ." When we learn that submitting means yielding ourselves to another, we can practice humility in a way that reinforces freedom.

THE IMPORTANCE AND IMPACT OF ACCOUNTABILITY

We see in 1 Peter 5:5 (NLT) how important it is to be accountable to each other: "All of you, dress yourselves in humility as you relate to one another, for 'God opposes the proud but gives grace to the humble.'" We must drop our pride and be humble enough to learn from other Christians who have walked the path a little longer or in different ways.

We also need to be bold enough to call other Christians out on their sin and ask why they are choosing to live in a way that goes against God's Word. We must be careful not to approach them in a way that implies we have any right to judge their behavior but in an understanding way. We need to clearly communicate that when one part of the body does something, the rest of the body is affected (1 Corinthians 12:26). It's important to have a genuine concern for the wellbeing of rebellious Christians; if you are more concerned with their behavior than their heart, then you are most likely not the one to approach them. Bring them to God in prayer and let God be God in that situation.

When holding someone accountable, the most important thing is to ask God for wisdom, discernment, and direction. Here's a hint: Get your own accountability with God and others in place first and it will be easier to recognize when you need to step out and hold someone else accountable. If you have no one holding you accountable for something, it may be time to step back and take a fresh look at pride and humility within your heart.

Accountability provides a safe place to grow in Christ and allow God to prune out the things in us that damage the kingdom of God and keep us walking in darkness. 1 Thessalonians 5:11 says, "Therefore encourage one another and build each other up, just as in fact you are doing." If we humble ourselves and allow God to grow us up in areas He reveals through other members in the body of Christ, we will become more like Christ and be more available for God to use us.

When it comes to our idolatry with emotional eating, the reality is that we have spent many years reinforcing these patterns of behavior. It's unrealistic to think we will overcome this stronghold overnight. How many times do you feel frustrated that this journey is taking too long? I understand that frustration and have to remind myself that I can't do this alone, and the more I try to, the longer this process will take.

My mentor, counselor, and close accountability partners have been so important in getting me where I am. God has used them to grow me up in spiritual truths I was struggling to hold onto, and they held me to my word while reminding me God was faithful to His when it came to making decisions I needed to make. Who, specifically, can you share your struggle with and ask to hold you accountable? What could this relationship of accountability with a sister or brother in Christ look like? In what ways will you be held accountable?

Remember, humility not only means we have a teachable spirit with our brothers and sisters in Christ, but it also means we have integrity. Integrity is being congruent internally with what we say externally. I need to have integrity with myself first and not play games. If I say I want to be held accountable to change, then I need to act like it — especially when no one is looking. When my accountability partner asks me how I've done with food this week, I must have integrity with her and not lie, otherwise what's the purpose of meeting for accountability anyway?

1 Thessalonians 5:14 says, "And we urge you, brothers and sisters, warn those who are idle and disruptive, encourage the disheartened, help the weak, be patient with everyone." Ultimately, as we hold each other accountable, we are to warn, encourage, and help those who are idle or undisciplined, discouraged, and weak. Above all, we are to be patient with one another. Of course, we can't forget to affirm others for their victories along the way. Always remember that we are not the Holy Spirit, so leave the convicting up to God, but we are to help one another live a life that reflects the grace, mercy, and freedom we have received from Christ.

SHIFTING GEARS

I love driving cars with a manual transmission. I don't know what it is about "stick shifts" that I love so much. Maybe it's the feeling that I have more control over my vehicle.

When driving up or down a hill, I often downshift to a lower gear. My engine has the same amount of power no matter what gear I'm in, but when I shift gears, my transmission adjusts how it locks the gears in place to cooperate with the engine and provide more specific help to carry the load and get me to my destination.

My dad drove large semitrucks for years and experienced not only the importance but also the necessity of downshifting. Depending on the grade of the hill, he would sometimes have to downshift through several gears. If he hadn't, the truck could have stalled out while going uphill or careened downhill out of control — especially if weather conditions were bad.

His vehicle wouldn't have been able to transport its large load successfully and safely.

It would be great for our engines if there were no hills, and you might feel the same about your life. But because there are ups and downs in this journey of overcoming emotional eating, we need to practice downshifting. Hard circumstances are like bad weather conditions—making the hills of this battle even more of a struggle. We can't coast through life on cruise control and expect to overcome strongholds. We must apply detailed attention and energy to put specific goals into action. Here are some examples of downshifting actions:

- Bible study time

- accountability meetings

- exercising

- food prepping

- grocery shopping

- understanding nutrition

- adjusting actions within trigger zones

No matter what, we have the same amount of power from the Holy Spirit, but by downshifting, we cooperate with the Holy Spirit who will continue to carry us throughout our freedom journey. Prayer helps us downshift, and as we are getting ready to plan meals, grocery shop, exercise, etc., we can use prayer as one of our weapons to dig deeper and keep climbing.

GET SMART

It's so easy to say, "I'm going to lose weight this week," or, "I'm going to go to the gym more this week," but since there is no structure to this type of goal, it can quickly fall to the wayside. Setting SMART (specific, measurable, attainable, relevant, time-sensitive) goals is a great tool to help reach milestones and gain ground when trying to overcome obstacles in our lives. SMART goals will help us stay accountable as we take what we've learned and apply it.

Keep in mind that setting goals is important, but without accountability to make sure we are reaching those goals, it can be hard to continue achieving the benchmarks along the way. We talked about the importance of accountability and how it can shape our success. If you're tempted to skip that step, remind yourself how well doing things on your own has worked out so far. I know for me, my struggle with food isolated me due to shame, guilt, and frustration. That isolation kept me struggling alone. Now, through accountability, I've met new benchmarks and won new ground. The journey continues.

Take time to set some goals. Organize them into three main categories: spiritual, mental-emotional, and physical. Be sure to create goals that follow the SMART format. Now that you have some goals in place—who will be your accountability partner? Give this person a copy of these goals and ask them to hold you accountable. Remember—the battle is never won alone.

Here are some ways to be accountable to each other:

- Text "negotiating" when you're in the negotiation process—after you've been triggered and before you eat. This gives the opportunity for your accountability partner to pray with and for you as well as speak some solid truth that helps you not give in and emotionally eat.

- Pray with each other.

- Study the Bible together.

- Visit a counselor. Report visits to your accountability partner.

- Make godly friendships that point you to Christ. Keep your accountability partner informed about the new friendships for prayer and guidance.

- Stay honest in your conversations.

- Build a mentorship relationship. Pray for God to bring you a mentor to learn from and then pray for someone to mentor when the timing is right.

- Join a Tenacious Grace Support Group.

- Hire a Tenacious Grace Coach to keep you accountable and help you along your journey.

"WOULD YOU LIKE TO TRY A SAMPLE?"

Let's tackle one major downshifting activity and talk about grocery shopping. How we shop in the grocery store is important — it will either set us up for success or failure.

For the emotional eater, grocery stores are a battlefield. We can't walk in without armor, the Holy Spirit's self-control, and a good shopping list. As a part of the emotional eating cycle, we learned how our senses play a big part in the trigger phase. Sight is a contributor to emotional eating. If we see everything as we walk down every aisle, how can we expect ourselves not to give in to temptation? We smell the food cooking over in the deli and, of course, don't forget about the lovely sample stands set up around the store with bite-size snacks that are waiting to engage with our taste buds. Oh, those things are so sneaky. I mean, how many times are you going to have a sample and *not* buy the entire bag?

If you are an aisle-browser without a list, you're more likely to buy comfort food than fuel. Walking the perimeter of the store (where most of the healthier and fresher foods are placed) and going straight to what's on your list are keys to a successful shopping trip. Lists not only limit emotional buying, but they also help your budget stay on track. Put work into your lists and see how successful you can be.

I remember being a kid and shopping with my mom at our local grocery store. I would hold the calculator and put in the price as she picked each food item off the shelf and placed it in our basket. She had a detailed list of which food items were in which aisle because she knew that if she was going to stick to her plan, she had to be intentional about it. Oh, the countless number of times I've failed to stick to plans that I didn't put much effort into. No wonder they didn't work.

When buying food, you also need to look at the ingredients. This is an aspect of stewardship where we take responsibility for what we put in our bodies. Check food labels and choose healthier options. If you feel that you'll be deprived if you don't get the junk food option, it's an emotional buy. Emotional purchases lead to emotional eating. Remind yourself food is fuel, and the healthier option will provide better fuel for your body.

SMART SHOPPING

I'd like to show you how to break down grocery shopping into the SMART goals process. This will give you a general idea of how I go about doing this, and then you can make it your own.

Make it Specific

I know that grocery shopping is my overall goal, but to make that specific, I write down the following:

Go to the grocery store and get the following:

- Almond Milk
- Orange Juice
- Eggs
- Salad
- Chips

- Salsa
- Sweet potatoes
- Zucchini
- Apples
- Chocolate covered almonds

You get the picture! The idea is to be as detailed as possible about the store and each item. If you have a budget you need to stay within, do your research on coupons, sales, and stores that will help you save money.

Make it Measurable

This answers the question, "How will I know I was successful in reaching my goal?" I like to leave a buffer of $10 *or* three extra items that weren't on my list. I know I will get to the store and see something I forgot I needed.

So, here is the way I make my grocery shopping goal measurable:

- If I come home with no more than three extra items or $10 above budget, I will know it was a successful trip.

Make it Attainable

This answers the question, "How will I plan to make this goal happen?" I know that if I shop on an empty stomach, I'm setting myself up for failure. I have to block time out of my schedule so that I'm not going to the store hungry.

Here is how I will attain my goal:

- Go to the grocery store on Friday morning after your training session and before work. Get a post-workout smoothie so you're not hungry while shopping.

Make it Relevant

When I'm setting goals, I'm easily distracted by multitasking. I tend to look at how much time I have and try to fit in as many things as I can instead of looking at what I need to do and planning my time around that. For instance, I could get off track by planning three or four other errands around my trip to the grocery store.

So I ask myself, "Are the S, M, and A sections relevant to my overarching goal?" For example, returning a purchase to a retail store down the road isn't relevant to my grocery shopping. Too many times to count, I've overloaded my to-do list with so many irrelevant stops that grocery shopping falls to the wayside. I've learned to plan time around grocery shopping and make that the only thing I do so I can be successful at it.

The relevant section of my goal looks like this:

- Run errands on Saturday morning, not Friday. On Friday, only go to the gym, get a smoothie, and then head to the grocery store.

Make it Time-Sensitive

We get stressed by the things we have left to do—not the things we get done. The first leaves us feeling overwhelmed and worried, and the second leaves us feeling productive and ready to take on the rest of our to-do list. Thinking through the time sensitivity of grocery shopping is important because we don't want to feel rushed, but we don't want to have too much time to browse and fall into the emotional buying trap.

Planning your shopping trip between appointments may be a good idea because it gives you a healthy sense of urgency that helps you get in, follow your list, and get out.

Here's how I can make my grocery shopping goal time-sensitive:

- Go to the gym from 8 to 9

- Get a smoothie between 9 and 9:20

- Only shop at the grocery store from 9:30 to 10:00 (30 minutes—in and out!)

Once I have my grocery shopping SMART goal written down, I give it to my accountability partner and have her hold me true to my plan. This is just one goal of many you can put through the SMART goal process. I encourage you to do so and bring your accountability partner in on it with you. We can't expect to change old habits without the help of others.

GOING DEEPER

1. Who will your accountability partner be? If you don't know, write some names of those you can be praying about. Then ask someone to keep you accountable through this journey.

2. What will you ask your partner to hold you accountable for? What measures of success will you put in place to ensure that accountability?

3. What SMART goals will you fight to accomplish?

OWNING TRUTH

- Accountability provides a safe place to grow in Christ and allow God to prune away the things in us that damage the kingdom of God and keep us walking in darkness.

- Goals that are specific, measurable, attainable, relevant, and time-sensitive are more likely to be accomplished than one general, overarching goal.

- Be intentional in the grocery store. Look at labels and come prepared with a plan so you stay on task.

CHAPTER 11

My Choice Button
Is Not Broken

Now that we've been intentional in letting God show us the *why* behind our emotional eating, it's time to start doing things differently. Exercise and nutrition are essential parts of a healthy lifestyle and can help us manage our newly redefined relationship with food.

STRONGER THAN YOU THINK

I was ten years old and in gym class getting ready for a pull-up. I had always been able to hoist my body up and down with the strength of my arms, but not that day. I clearly remember feeling my strength betray me and leave me there, hanging and grunting in front of my classmates as I tried to pull myself up.

After that, I identified as someone who didn't have any upper body strength. I accepted it and laughed it off while secretly admiring women who could do pull-ups.

For the last few years, I've been meeting with a personal trainer and lifting weights. I have found a new love for weight-lifting and feeling strong. What I've learned as I've pushed myself to pick up more and more weight and build muscle is that I actually do have a strong upper body. As I increased my workout weight on the bench press and shoulder press, my inner ten-year-old was consistently shocked. I heard God whisper to my heart so many times during my workouts, "See, you're physically stronger than you think you are. Imagine how much stronger you can be spiritually because of My power in you."

I would never have learned my true strength if I hadn't put in the work. God created our bodies to move and to work. Genesis 2:15 says, "The Lord God took the man and put him in the garden of Eden to work it and take care of it." From the start, human beings were physically active. While desk jobs are a part of the culture we live in, and there's nothing wrong with having a desk job, wisdom tells us to make exercise a priority in our lives. If I sit at work all day, go home to sit, sleep, then do it all over again, I'm not stewarding my body the way God told me to.

Let's look at some benefits of exercise. An incredibly effective way to lose weight is to burn more calories than you consume. Exercise helps maintain healthy weight levels by increasing the number of calories burned. This works as long as our emotional eating is under control and the number of calories we're consuming is similar to the number we burn. When we exercise, blood flows better and regulates the cholesterol in our heart. Exercise helps prevent or manage cardiovascular diseases, metabolic syndrome, type 2 diabetes, depression, certain types of cancer, and more.

Another great result of exercise is that it boosts your mood by stimulating brain chemicals (neurotransmitters such as dopamine, oxytocin, and endorphins) that help you feel better. It also boosts energy levels by delivering oxygen and nutrients to your tissues, which helps your heart and lungs work more efficiently. Other benefits like better sleep and an enhanced sexual drive also come from exercise. God designed us to move, and thankfully, it comes with benefits!

Exercising when we don't want to is an outward expression of an inward commitment: a commitment to put our immediate desires to the side. We need to value longevity of health as a great reward and a part of presenting our bodies as living sacrifices to the Lord. The long-term benefits are worth the momentary sacrifice.

It's almost guaranteed that, at first, we won't be exercise experts. When will we put excuses to death? When will we do what we can even if we don't reach our ideal? When will we allow ourselves the ability to improve? We can't improve on something we never start. Is our undisciplined exercise a reflection of the way we make excuses for not spending time in the Word and doing spiritual and emotional exercises throughout each day? Colossians 3:23–24 (BSB) tells us, "Whatever you do, work at it with your whole being, for the Lord and not for men, because you know that you will receive an inheritance from the Lord as your reward. It is the Lord Christ you are serving." Let's get moving, learn how to fuel our bodies, and make one small step toward change each day!

FOOD AS FUEL

We need food to be the energy our bodies can burn daily for activities as well as when we are exercising. When trying to create healthy eating habits, it's easy to get overwhelmed by all the contradictory research, diets, and programs out there. Which is better: vegan, paleo, vegetarian, pescatarian, or keto? Should we be eating a high-carb, raw, or starch-based diet? Do you eat before or after a workout? What do you eat for pre or post workout meals? I'm not going to direct you toward one specific way of eating. Whichever type of healthy eating lifestyle you want to choose, you have my blessing, as long as you're within the boundaries of eating for fuel and not for an emotional fix.

Many people are passionate about their healthy eating lifestyle of choice, and they want to argue about nutrition and convince others to eat the same way they do. Their diet has worked for them, so it's natural they think it's the only way. We must be careful about this. One can easily adopt a belief system that judges others for their food choices. Different diets work for different people's bodies. The most important thing is whether or not the position of one's heart and will is that of stewardship and honoring God or that of idolatry.

In Romans 14:13, 17, Paul says, "Therefore let us stop passing judgment on one another. Instead, make up your mind not to put any stumbling block or obstacle in the way of a brother or sister. ... For the kingdom of God is not a matter of eating and drinking, but of righteousness, peace and joy in the Holy Spirit." When we get caught up in the debate about which healthy lifestyle is best, we put the focus on food again instead of the heart.

We are not here to cause each other to stumble. We let others have their conviction on what they believe is best for their body and trust God to reveal new truth if He sees it's necessary. Please seek out a nutritionist or do some research and learn, on a basic biological level, what food does when you ingest it. I don't claim to be a doctor or nutritionist, so I won't go into all the nutrition lessons I've learned, but I will tell you that learning what food does in my body has helped tremendously in my journey of overcoming emotional eating.

If you join a Tenacious Grace Support Group, you'll learn about how nutrients are broken down. Learning about the biological breakdown of food helps to see the reality of the harmful effects in our bodies from the food we're eating. This removes more of the power we've placed on food to meet our needs. If you hire a Tenacious Grace Coach, you'll get a personalized approach to how the foods you eat effect your body and how that impacts your daily activities. For more information about joining a group, becoming a group facilitator, hiring a coach, or becoming a certified Tenacious Grace Coach, please reference the appendices at the back of this book.

ONE SIZE DOESN'T FIT ALL

Our God is a God of balance, and He tells us in Ecclesiastes 7:16–18 to avoid extremes. We need to always keep in mind that we are to strive for a balanced lifestyle of eating, one that reflects a heart that's positioned toward worshipping God and not food. When our hearts are in this surrendered position, we will make choices about food that reflect a decision to eat for health and fuel.

What works for one won't necessarily work for all, and this is where we put Romans 14:13 into practice. Focus on learning about what you're putting in your body—what it does in your body, and if it's important for your body's needs—and quit worrying about what someone else is doing with their food choices.

Whenever I'm struggling to stick with a healthy lifestyle, I find it easy to go into "control mode." I'll get on a brand new diet, do a cleanse or fast, change up my workout routine—I mean, I can come up with some crazy plans to lose weight fast. That, my friend, is why I wrote this book. These control tactics are a sign that we are turning to *how* answers for our *why* questions. Yes, they help. Yes, they have their place. But if they are what we turn to first, we will forever be caught up in the emotional eating cycle.

You may go on a crash diet and lose weight, but when the next big life change comes along, you'll be right back here. My goal is that you will learn to have a balanced relationship with food—one where you view it as fuel for your body and not a fix for your heart—and address the root of the matter first.

I hope you focus on the truths shared in this book, truths God has revealed to you throughout your healing journey, and you will reposition your heart to get off the throne and put God in His rightful place.

Here is what gets me back on track when my eating feels out of control: I stay within the pocket of what I know to be true. This means I have a clear set of principles and truth to live by regarding food and when I'm in the pocket, I'm not wavering from those. Whenever I feel out of control, I know I need to return to truth and those principles. I intentionally recite them to help me return to truth.

This is my truth pocket: Food cannot and will not meet my heart's needs. Food is food. Food is fuel. God, however, can and will meet and fulfill my heart's every need to overflowing.

These are my principles:

1. Feast on God's Word.

2. Only eat to fuel my body.

3. Outsmart emotional cravings.

4. Decide to eat nutritious foods.

I pray that this will help you to remember to deal with the position of your heart first. Discover the *why* behind your emotional eating before trying to implement the *how* of interacting differently with food.

WHO WILL IT BE?

Every time you choose to emotionally eat, you also choose to say no to God. The opposite can be true — every time you turn to God for your emotional or spiritual needs, you say no to emotional eating. Now, at your crossroads moment, there is a big sign ahead of you that says, "Do differently!" The choice is yours to make. I can't make it for you (believe me, I wish I could be your pocket-sized Tenacious Grace Coach), but if you have been saved by grace through faith in Jesus Christ, you have the Holy Spirit to guide you and sisters and brothers in Christ to hold you accountable. You have the best source of strength to make new choices and walk in a new way. You can redefine your relationship with food — enjoy it without letting it be your emotional fix.

Answer this honestly: Are you going to continue to only talk about and be frustrated by your emotional eating issues, or are you going to start doing things differently, believing in faith that God will bring you out of this as you follow Him in obedience?

Choose who you will serve, as Joshua did in Joshua 24:14–15. He put the challenge out to his people to stop serving other gods and choose to worship and serve only the true God. Joshua told the Israelites that he was moving ahead toward the blessings of God in his life and his family's lives with or without them, and if they wanted to take part in the blessings of God, they would need to be intentional and draw a line in the sand — choosing to follow God in action as well as speech. The people chose to serve God alongside Joshua. The Israelites and Joshua then set up some accountability markers with new rules and parameters because of their new commitment to each other and God. Through this decision, accountability, and community, they had to learn to redefine their relationship with the many false gods of their time and redirect their worship to the one true God.

A verse that humbles me every time that I am reminded I need to make a choice is 1 Corinthians 10:21 (NLT). It says, "You cannot drink from the cup of the Lord and from the cup of demons, too. You cannot eat at the Lord's Table and at the table of demons, too." I get a visual picture of two tables with a cup on each. Imagine with me one table is filled with Satan's demons who seek to deceive us with lies of idolatry, gluttony, power, and control. The other is our powerful yet tender love, Jesus who seeks to heal, protect, bless, and love us. Food, when not in its rightful place, can be a tool in Satan's hands to keep us from a thriving love relationship with Jesus. Friend, choose the table with Jesus – He is the Bread of Life and the Living Water. Nothing is more satisfying to our hearts than Him.

GOING DEEPER

1. What does your outward commitment level to exercising reflect about your inward commitment to choosing a healthier lifestyle?

2. Do you compare your healthy eating habits to those of other people who eat healthily? If so, does that help or hurt your progress?

3. When you can't seem to get your emotional eating under control, do you stop and adjust the position of your heart? If not, write out a prayer that will help you change position from one of idolatry with food to one of surrender to God.

OWNING TRUTH

• Start with small changes like adding in one workout a week and changing one unhealthy habit with your food. Don't seek out perfection, but rather commit to perseverance.

• The healthier we eat, the easier exercise gets! God created our bodies to move, and He made food to fuel them.

• Joshua told the Israelites to choose which god they would serve. God is asking you to choose today. Who will you serve: God or food?

Conclusion

Let's look back at what we've learned through this journey and grasp the big picture. God is tenacious in His pursuit of our hearts. He longs for us to be satisfied by Him alone, and He longs to be gracious to us. His grace means He is good to us and shows us favor. God gives us the power of the Holy Spirit to overcome strongholds and walk in right relationship with Him—where we get our emotional security from Him rather than food.

Defining the specific relationship we have with food is where we need to start. We have triggers, and it's vitally important to be aware of what they are. We have to find the starting point where our thoughts and feelings lead us to certain types of food. Understanding these patterns helps us recognize why we struggle and what exactly we are looking for in food. A part of the struggle is that food means something more to us than fuel: comfort, companionship, escape, etc. We must spend the time to understand how we have attached to food emotionally.

At its core, emotional eating is idolatry. Idolatry is exchanging the truth about God for a lie, worshipping and serving created things rather than the Creator. Idols don't give—they take from us. Idolatry is driven by pride, it distorts our reality, and it reinforces faulty relationship dependency. We turn to

151

food when we think we know what serves our hearts' needs better than God does, but idolatry will always cost us something.

Identifying the type of hunger we're experiencing helps to break the emotional eating cycle. Spiritual, emotional, and physical hunger are the three types of hunger present in our lives. If we haven't learned to know the difference, we will by default turn to food to satisfy them all. Being prepared by knowing what to feed each type of hunger will help us move forward confidently in each area.

Emotional hunger starts with our thought patterns — the unhealthy ones that we don't identify and tend to create emotions we may not be aware of. When we're in this state, our feelings are in the driver's seat. We must do the mental work to refocus our thoughts and the spiritual work to put truth in the driver's seat.

Physical hunger has physiological symptoms. We need to give ourselves enough time between meals to recognize our bodies' signals and fuel them with food that will help us grow stronger and healthier.

Spiritual hunger occurs when we haven't gone to our Creator to fulfill our hearts as only He can. We keep turning to food, wanting it to fill our hearts when it doesn't have the power to do so.

To stop the momentum of the emotional eating cycle we need to live intentionally and not get stuck on autopilot. Intentional living is where we fight the thoughts this life throws at us that become triggers. We must use prayer, truth, and accountability to analyze our thoughts, annihilate the lies from Satan, and then appropriate the truth from Jesus. We learn to replace lies with truth and walk in freedom.

We negotiate with Satan too long and get caught in the emotional eating cycle of the trigger, eating, and shame phases. If we live out of balance, our responses will be out of balance. We tend to operate in the urgency of the body's fight or flight response due to our busyness and anxiety, which tears us down physically and emotionally. It's important to carve out time for our bodies to activate the rest and digest system so they can refresh and repair. These times also keep our minds steady and focused on the truth. When we are in the rest and digest mode, we are less likely to binge on food or choose unhealthy foods when we are not hungry.

The emotional eating cycle starts when we are triggered, so we need to be aware of what's going on around us and be alert and sober-minded, as the Bible tells us in 1 Peter 5:8. The things we focus on and the thoughts we don't take captive will determine how we interact with food, so we must do our main fighting in the trigger phase. When we eat "feeling foods" when we aren't hungry, our senses are engaged in the sight, sound, taste, smell, and touch of the food, and we have a sense of euphoria. These senses act as triggers.

When we engage in emotional eating, it feels as though we have found the answer, but that feeling wears off quickly. We must learn to jam the firing pin of this mechanism of emotional eating and recognize when we are triggered so we can put truth in place and turn to God instead. Just because we started eating, doesn't mean we can't put the food down and break the cycle.

After emotionally eating, we tend to wallow in the shame phase, where Satan throws guilt on us like a weighted blanket of despair. We realize the emotional eating phase wasn't all it was built up to be during the trigger phase, and what we're left with is another blow to our already low self-esteem. Satan uses shame as a tool to trick us into looking at ourselves differently. We overcome shame by spiritually fighting back, humbling ourselves before the Lord, appropriating Jesus' righteousness, memorizing His truths, and clinging to the truth that God is enthralled and captivated by our beauty.

Our sins had a price that only Jesus could pay. Jesus died to set us free because we couldn't pay the price then, and we can't now. That's why we rely on grace to sustain us as we do our best to honor God and walk in obedience. God approves of us because He sees His Son's blood covering our sins which makes us righteous and in good standing with God. The stronghold of emotional eating keeps tripping us up because it's a false belief system where we seek shelter to escape reality of unmet heart desires. We believe that we're powerless when, in truth, we are powerful warriors who can overcome these strongholds through the power of Christ and the weapons of warfare He gives us.

We must consistently remind ourselves of Romans 8:11, which tells us we have *full* access to the power of God that raised Jesus from the dead: the Holy Spirit who lives within us. We are rich in righteousness, and it's time we act like it. We can claim that righteousness by putting on our spiritual armor, using the weapons of spiritual warfare, and *choosing* to fight even if we don't feel like it. We have the belt of truth, breastplate of righteousness, helmet of salvation, shield of faith, shoes of the gospel of peace, sword of God's truth, a cloak of zeal, and prayer as armor and weapons to activate that power in our lives.

Accountability plays a huge role in how we succeed in this battle. Getting outside ourselves and acting as a member of the body of Christ will help us realize that when we worship food and ourselves, it affects other believers. It takes vulnerability and humility with our brothers and sisters in Christ to remain accountable.

Having some structure to our accountability efforts in the form of setting some SMART goals will help us gain more ground. To implement our goals and the things we've learned through this journey, we must pray and seek God first — above all else.

Managing a newly redefined relationship with food calls for us to do differently in two areas: exercise and nutrition. Exercising provides opportunities to implement intentional discipline of our bodies through an external commitment that reflects our inward desire to be healthier all around. Our bodies were created to be active. Food can no longer be seen as a comfort, companion, or escape. We need to see it as fuel for our bodies on a biological level. We need to eat healthy food that gives us the most benefits. No singular way of eating works for everyone; the important thing is to stay consistent.

We need to put one foot in front of the other and keep walking this different path. It will all click into place as we keep moving forward, and we will eventually walk more consistently in freedom. One step at a time, one meal at a time . . . we keep moving forward.

EYES ON THE PRIZE

Paul tells us in Philippians 3:13–14 (ESV), "But one thing I do: forgetting what lies behind and straining forward to what lies ahead, I press on toward the goal for the prize of the upward call of God in Christ Jesus." We must forget the failures behind us and focus on the victories we've had along the journey.

There are greater victories to be won ahead. Keep pressing on. Today is the day to make your choice. Who will you serve? I am choosing to serve God. I know I won't be perfect at it and I can't measure success by the state of my body, but rather the position of my heart. The body changes will follow in time as I stay consistently surrendered to God's way of engaging with food, not mine. Although I will mess up along the way, that doesn't give me the excuse to not fight with all I have to press into the power of the Holy Spirit and let Him change me from the inside out. I'm going forward with or without you, but I would love to have you with me! Don't allow your emotional appetite for food to be your false god and stop you from joining others in experiencing a deeper level of freedom and intimacy with Jesus.

Besides Joshua, there's another man in the Bible who called his people to make a choice. Elijah was sick and tired of the idolatry that had run rampant throughout his country. He called out the false prophets for a showdown. In 1 Kings 18:21–39, you can read how he chose to battle 850 prophets of the false gods Baal and Asherah in front of the people of Israel.

I love verse 21 (ESV) where Elijah asks the people, "How long will you go limping between two different opinions? If the Lord is God, follow him; but if Baal, then follow him." Elijah was calling out the people of Israel as much as he was the false prophets. A choice needed to be made for God's people to truly claim their freedom and walk in it.

The word "limping" gives me a great picture of what it feels like when I go back and forth between the idolatry of emotional eating and the obedience of eating for fuel. Only when I choose to fight time after time do I get stronger in the battle. I may feel like a bruised-up mess, but at least I'm not limping in those moments. I'm standing firm.

Elijah chose to follow God and challenged the false prophets to a show of power from their gods. He set up specific parameters for how the showdown between the false gods—Baal and Asherah—and the one true God—Jehovah, God of Abraham, Isaac, and Jacob—would happen. He told the prophets to get a bull and place it on an altar, and he would do the same. But the wood for the sacrifices was not to be lit with fire. The true God would be the one who consumed His bull with fire from the heavens.

Elijah gave the false prophets a shot at it first. Sadly for the prophets, Baal and Asherah didn't deliver, even after the false prophets began cutting themselves and doing everything they could think to call down the power of their gods.

At the end of the day, it was Elijah's turn. You know he was itching for those final moments when God would get the glory and allow him to watch the false prophets squirm. God told Elijah to rebuild a broken altar (verse 30) and set the stage for God to show His true power.

God came through for Elijah and revealed that He is the one true God, and He did so with flair. God told Elijah to make the circumstances seem impossible for the sacrifice to be consumed by fire, drenching it with gallons of water three times—filling a trench surrounding the altar. God then consumed the sacrifice of the bull by fire that fell from heaven. Not only was the bull consumed, but the altar itself and even the water in the trench were as well.

How many times do we act like these false prophets, hurting our bodies through binging on poor quality foods or not eating at all? We do those things to call down the power of food to meet our emotional or spiritual needs. Baal and Asherah held no power, and neither does the food we eat.

I love that God chose a broken altar. Every time we commit idolatry with food, we break the altar of sacrifice where God calls us to deny ourselves, pick up our cross, and follow Him. But every time we worship God and not food, we are rebuilding that broken altar for God to show His power and consume our sacrifice.

Our circumstances may seem impossible for God to come through and accept our offering of worship, but God works best in impossible circumstances. Matthew 19:26 tells us that with God, all things are possible — including overcoming emotional eating. Without God, the false prophets' sacrifice was not consumed by fire; *with* God, Elijah's was.

Who are you going to continue to serve: the idols of self and food or the one true God? Food cannot and will not deliver what we want because it is not God. Food is food. Food is fuel for our bodies. It holds no power emotionally or spiritually. God is calling us to rebuild a broken altar within our hearts. As we present ourselves as living sacrifices through a healthy relationship with food, He is faithful to show up and consume that sacrifice. Give God the opportunity to prove His faithfulness and power to bring you out of this stronghold. Obedience to God's truth sets the stage for His power!

Lord Jesus, thank You for the gift of grace that You give us from Your redemptive choice to follow God in obedience and sacrifice Yourself on the cross. Thank You that through this gift, we can have eternal life and a relationship with God through You. Thank You for Your truth through Your Word and Your Holy Spirit.

Father God, I come before You in Jesus' name, thankful that through a relationship with Jesus, I am able to ask You for an extra dose of power, protection, revelation of truth, and blessing over the ones reading this book and walking this journey. Please bless them as they walk their own freedom journey.

*In Jesus' name and with the authority given to me as one of
God's daughters, I come up against the influence of Satan and
his lies, intimidation, and manipulation in these dear lives.
I claim truth for their minds, protection for their hearts, and
freedom for their lives — that their stronghold with food will be
shattered and the only refuge they run to is Jesus Christ!*

*God, I ask that the truths learned here permeate the far corners
of their minds and hearts. I pray they would come to know You
personally and enter into a relationship with You if they haven't
already. I also pray they would become trained and mighty warriors in the battle of identifying and overcoming idolatry.*

*Jesus, I love You so much and am beyond humbled and grateful
for You and my own freedom journey. Thank You for honoring
me by using my pain and my surrender to impact these dear
lives through this book.
In Jesus' name, I pray this. Amen.*

Please reach out to me, as I would love to know your journeys,
struggles, and victories. My contact information is in the back
of this book along with extra resources.

Dear heart, you have been prayed over, fought for, and are
being pursued by God Almighty, the One who created you.
It's time — stop running to food and start running to God. Then
keep running to Him over and over again.

Appendix I

TAKE YOUR NEXT STEPS AND DON'T DO IT ALONE!

Join a Tenacious Grace Support Group

Changing years of unhealthy emotional attachments to food is hard. It's even harder if you're doing it alone.

When you're a part of a Tenacious Grace Support Group, you can relate to others in the ups and downs of the journey to overcome emotional eating. You can find strength and encouragement from other overcomers walking alongside you. Your group can be a powerful resource in redefining your relationship with food.

Visit www.tenaciousgracejourney.com for more information and to find a group near you.

Hire a Tenacious Grace Coach

How many times have you wished you had someone to help you overcome something step by step? Sometimes you need one-on-one guidance to take you deeper into the exploration of what causes you to emotionally eat.

With Tenacious Grace Coaching, you will find a coach who is passionate about helping you redefine your relationship with food. You'll have direct access to your coach for sessions, encouragement, and accountability.

It's time to go the extra step and receive the individualized help you've been hoping for.

Visit www.tenaciousgracejourney.com to find out more information and hire your coach.

Join the tribe!

Join the conversation on Facebook and become a part of the online community at www.facebook.com/tenaciousgraceTG

PERSONAL TESTIMONIES

I have struggled with emotional eating for as long as I can remember. My weight fluctuated through the years, but I was able to keep my weight within a healthy range. However, in 2012 I was blessed to become pregnant with our son. I gained 70+ pounds while pregnant and on bed rest. A few pounds were shed before becoming pregnant with our daughter. I gained another 50+ pounds with my second pregnancy — yikes! Motherhood is an absolute dream come true, however, my daily struggle with emotional eating was robbing me of joy.

Through attending the Tenacious Grace Support Groups, my relationship with food has changed and my understanding of God's Word with regard to this stronghold has grown.

Thanks to Jenna and *Tenacious Grace*, my mind and heart have been transformed. Jenna's heart for the Lord and others, as well as her knowledge of God's Word and how it applies to our lives, is clearly evident in this book and the workbook used in the groups. For anyone struggling with emotional eating, I highly recommend joining a group. Tenacious Grace Support Groups have been truly life changing.

— **Mary**, St. Louis, Missouri

Starting in fifth grade, I began to hold an infatuation with the food I was consuming — or rather, what I was ceasing to consume. Restriction quickly became a game that I played in order to watch myself become something different in the mirror instead of allowing my mind to thrive. My unhealthy relationship with food became unhealthy relationships with men, friends, family, and an overall distaste for the life I had ahead of me.

Through Tenacious Grace Coaching, I have learned immense amounts of truth that have aided in the process of recovery from an overly restrictive mindset. It has become a toolbox that I leave open 24/7 in order to continue reminding myself that I have immeasurable worth in Christ. I have been taught that I am fully loved, known, and wanted by the One far greater than me—that He has created me as His masterpiece.

I would encourage anyone struggling with food to check out the wonderful guidance found in Tenacious Grace Coaching. An unhealthy relationship with food will follow you, but a healthy relationship with Christ will lead you.

—**Julia**, St. Louis, Missouri

INSPIRE OTHERS TOWARD FREEDOM!

Lead a Tenacious Grace Support Group

Are you longing to help others end emotional eating? Would you enjoy leading a small group of people through the companion Tenacious Grace Workbook? This downloadable workbook will guide the conversation so you can dig deeper with group members to reach new levels of awareness and discovery along the journey. These groups can be formed in a home, church, organization, or at your favorite coffeehouse.

Visit www.tenaciousgracejourney.com for more information and to facilitate a support group.

Become a Certified Tenacious Grace Coach

Do you have a passion to see God's truth set people free? Have you overcome or are you currently putting the work in with your battle with food? Do you want to use your experience with emotional eating to inspire others to do the same?

If you said yes to any of those questions, then becoming a certified Tenacious Grace Coach is for you. Becoming certified allows you to build your own clientele of individuals who will hire you to walk alongside them in their efforts to redefine their relationship with food.

Visit www.tenaciousgracejourney.com to find out more and become certified as a coach.

Appendix II

DREAMING FOR THE FUTURE

Watch for a lineup of resources and events soon to be released for the Tenacious Grace tribe:

- Niche support groups specifically for moms, singles, women, men, teens, etc.

- Annual Tenacious Grace Live Conference

- Online courses taking you deeper with the different aspects of the Tenacious Grace journey

- Tenacious Grace Podcast

- Tenacious Grace daily devotional—short messages to help you stay focused on gaining freedom from emotional eating. It will address the question of how you can love your body in a God-glorifying way even as it's in need of healing and repair.

Your voice matters! Jenna would like to know how she and her team can best serve you.

Connect with us at www.tenaciousgracejourney.com and become a part of the online community at www.facebook.com/tenaciousgraceTG

Appendix III

BRING JENNA TO YOUR EVENT!

Speaker – Author – Counselor – Coach

Jenna's mission is to inspire resilience while leading others to the heart of Christ. Her vision is to take you on a journey through deeper exploration into what motivates your behaviors. She has a passion for inspiring women to become more confident in their faith and relationships. Some areas Jenna loves to speak on include the following:

- Emotional Eating
- Singleness
- Worth
- Identity
- Comparison
- Purity
- Esteem
- Conflict
- Relationships
- Family Dynamics

- Fear

- Anxiety

- Depression

- Suicide

Jenna has been speaking publicly for fifteen years. She brings a powerful testimony to whomever she serves with her experience of life's ups and downs, failures and victories, hurts and healing, but ultimately, finding freedom in Christ. She would be honored to speak at your next event.

Connect with her today at www.jennabarbosa.com.

About the Author

JENNA BARBOSA

Jenna is thriving as a single woman in her thirties who loves writing books and riding motorcycles. She inspires people all over the world to live unhindered by faulty belief systems.

Jenna is the founder of Tenacious Grace — a ministry that provides group support and individual coaching to those desiring to overcome emotional eating.

A speaker, certified biblical counselor, and life coach, Jenna is passionate about teaching biblical principles and values found in God's Word. These have not only changed her life but also the lives of many she has influenced.

Visit JennaBarbosa.com to learn more about Jenna.

Endnotes

1   "Tenacious | Definition of Tenacious in English by Oxford Dictionaries." Oxford Dictionaries | English. Accessed April 30, 2019. https://en.oxforddictionaries.com/definition/tenacious.

2   "Grace | Definition of Grace in English by Oxford Dictionaries." Oxford Dictionaries | English. Accessed April 30, 2019. https://en.oxforddictionaries.com/definition/grace.

3   Ibid.

4   "Personification | Definition of Personification in English by Oxford Dictionaries." Oxford Dictionaries | English. Accessed May 01, 2019. https://en.oxforddictionaries.com/definition/personification.

5   "Comfort Zone | Definition of Comfort Zone in English by Oxford Dictionaries." Oxford Dictionaries | English. Accessed May 04, 2019. https://en.oxforddictionaries.com/definition/comfort_zone.

6   Strong, James. "3806. Pathos." Bible Hub. Accessed May 04, 2019. https://biblehub.com/greek/3806.htm.

7   "Emotion | Definition of Emotion in English by Oxford Dictionaries." Oxford Dictionaries | English. Accessed May 07, 2019. https://en.oxforddictionaries.com/definition/emotion.

8   Penn M., Goldstein D.J. (2005) "The Role of Hunger and Satiety in Weight Management." In: Goldstein D.J. (eds) The Management of Eating Disorders and Obesity. Nutrition and Health. Humana Press

9   "Intentionality | Definition of Intentionality in English by Oxford Dictionaries." Oxford Dictionaries | English. Accessed May 07, 2019. https://en.oxforddictionaries.com/definition/intentionality.

10 "Analyse | Definition of Analyse in English by Oxford Dictionaries." Oxford Dictionaries | English. Accessed May 07, 2019. https://en.oxforddictionaries.com/definition/analyse.

11 "Trigger | Definition of Trigger in English by Oxford Dictionaries." Oxford Dictionaries | English. Accessed May 08, 2019. https://en.oxforddictionaries.com/definition/trigger.

12 "Device | Definition of Device in English by Oxford Dictionaries." Oxford Dictionaries | English. Accessed May 08, 2019. https://en.oxforddictionaries.com/definition/device.

13 "Mechanism | Definition of Mechanism in English by Oxford Dictionaries." Oxford Dictionaries | English. Accessed May 08, 2019. https://en.oxforddictionaries.com/definition/mechanism.

14 "Trauma | Definition of Trauma in English by Oxford Dictionaries." Oxford Dictionaries | English. Accessed May 08, 2019. https://en.oxforddictionaries.com/definition/trauma.

15 C Tou, Janet & Fitch, Cindy & Bridges, Kayla. (2011). "Sweeteners: Uses, dietary intake and health effects."

16 "Condemnation | Definition of Condemnation in English by Oxford Dictionaries." Oxford Dictionaries | English. Accessed May 13, 2019. https://en.oxforddictionaries.com/definition/condemnation.

17 Strong, James. "3794. Ochuróma." Bible Hub. Accessed May 14, 2019. https://biblehub.com/greek/3794.htm.

18 Strong, James. "5485. Charis." Bible Hub. Accessed May 14, 2019. https://biblehub.com/greek/5485.htm.

19 Strong, James. "2590. Karpos." Bible Hub. Accessed May 14, 2019. https://biblehub.com/greek/2590.htm.

20 Strong, James. "266. Hamartia." Bible Hub. Accessed May 15, 2019. https://biblehub.com/greek/266.htm.

21 Strong, James. "2961. "Kurieuó." Bible Hub. Accessed May 15, 2019. https://biblehub.com/greek/2961.htm.

22 "Zeal | Definition of Zeal in English by Oxford Dictionaries." Oxford Dictionaries | English. Accessed May 16, 2019. https://en.oxforddictionaries.com/definition/zeal.

23 "Accountable | Definition of Accountable in English by Oxford Dictionaries." Oxford Dictionaries | English. Accessed May 16, 2019. https://en.oxforddictionaries.com/definition/accountable.

Made in the USA
Monee, IL
21 July 2021